The Body "Knows"

Other Hay House Titles of Related Interest

Books

Heal Your Body A–Z, by Louise L. Hay

Holy Spirit for Healing, by Ron Roth, Ph.D.,
with Peter Occhiogrosso

Natural Mental Health, by Carla Wills-Brandon

The Reconnection: Heal Others, Heal Yourself, by Dr. Eric Pearl

Your Personality, Your Health, by Carol Ritberger, Ph.D.

Menopause Made Easy, by Carolle Jean-Murat, M.D.

Audio Programs

Body Talk, by Mona Lisa Schulz, M.D., Ph.D.,
and Christiane Northrup, M.D.

Healing Your Body, Mind, and Soul, by Sylvia Browne

Unleashing Your Own Psychic Potential, by John Edward

Wisdom of the Masters, by Dr. Wayne W. Dyer

—⟨⟩—

All of the above are available at your local bookstore,
or may be ordered through Hay House, Inc.:

(800) 654-5126 or **(760) 431-7695**
(800) 650-5115 (fax) or **(760) 431-6948 (fax)**
www.hayhouse.com

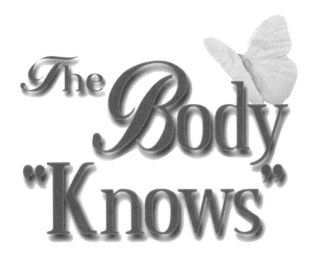

How to Tune In to Your Body and Improve Your Health

Caroline M. Sutherland

Hay House, Inc.
Carlsbad, California • Sydney, Australia

Published and distributed in the United States by:
Hay House, Inc., P.O. Box 5100, Carlsbad, CA 92018-5100
(800) 654-5126 • (800) 650-5115 (fax) • www.hayhouse.com

Editorial supervision: Jill Kramer • *Assistant editor:* Shannon Todd
Design: Summer McStravick

Library of Congress Cataloging-in-Publication Data

Sutherland, Caroline M.
 The body "knows" : how to tune in to your body and improve your health / Caroline M. Sutherland.
  p. cm.
 ISBN 1-56170-842-9
 1. Nutrition. 2. Intuition (Psychology) I. Title.

RA784 . S87 2001
613—dc21

00-065341

ISBN 1-56170-842-9

04 03 02 01   4 3 2 1
1st printing, September 2001

Printed in Canada

*To my father (the doctor) in heaven,
and to my mother, Mary*

Contents

PART IV: Tuning In to the Emotions and Spirit

PART V: Putting It All Together to Heal Your Family and Yourself

APPENDIX

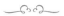

Please Note: All of the stories and case studies
in this book are true. All names have been
changed for confidentiality purposes.

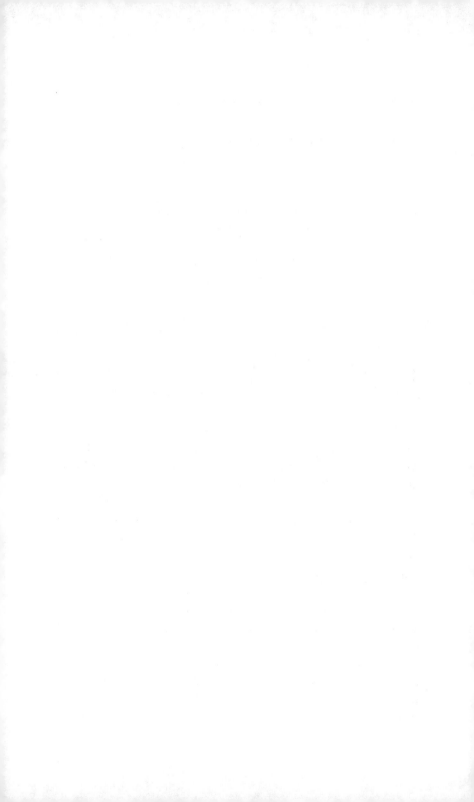

Foreword

by Julian Kenyon, M.D.

*"The natural healing force within each of us
is the greatest force in getting well."*
— Hippocrates

It is with great pleasure that I write this Foreword to Caroline Sutherland's most recent book. I've known Caroline for many years, and several years ago, I had the privilege of teaching her some of the modalities that are covered in *The Body "Knows."*

Caroline has had a varied life experience and many personal challenges, both of which have given her extraordinary wisdom. She has an infectious sense of enthusiasm and positivity about her, which comes across in this book.

Caroline gives a sensible view of medical intuition—she hasn't blinded the reader with science. *The Body "Knows"* deals with a whole range of approaches to tuning in to the body that anybody could implement at home. The information is presented in a simple and easily understandable way. The book also points out a variety of self-help approaches, dealing with a whole range of illnesses—and all of us are afflicted by these illnesses, to some extent, at various times in our lives. It is good to see a book that encourages these "natural" approaches and doesn't overmedicalize problems with conventional pharmaceuticals, which almost always carry a significant risk and a downside to them.

Overall, this book gives a view of how the body works in simple terms. Once we build on the basis of this understanding, it is possible to figure out a whole range of problems that may be affecting us, and to then come up with a reasonable solution. If none of these procedures work, then it is important to seek medical advice, but in the first instance, there is no doubt that one's own intuition (and the intuition of those close to us) is nearly always right. The medical profession in general tends to downplay listening to intuition, so I very much hope that this book will give the ordinary person more power and courage to listen to their own bodies and act accordingly. These "gifts" are so often disregarded by the medical profession, as they are not "scientific" in the medical sense. As a result, many doctors don't "listen" at all. Hopefully this book will empower the reader, *and* enable doctors to learn more from their patients. *The Body "Knows"* deserves a wide readership.

— Julian Kenyon, M.D., London, England
  www.doveclinic.com

Foreword

by Timothy Thar, M.D.

In the last 20 years, there have been dramatic changes in health care. In the past, the patient was usually a fairly passive participant in treatment decisions and was given little knowledge of the therapeutic options. Now, in increasing numbers, patients are taking more personal responsibility for their health. With the advent of the Internet, and much more readily available medical information, an increasing amount of patients are taking an active role in their treatment. If you're in this category, you might be interested in exploring and getting to know the wisdom of the body, which resides within you.

When I first met Caroline Sutherland, I was impressed with her insights, her vibrant health, and her passion to help people on their healing journeys. With loving compassion, she works with people to develop better health habits, drawing on her many years of experience as a medical intuitive. She is also a very capable teacher, helping people to connect with the inner healer in each of us.

My medical education in the early '70s was focused on learning treatment protocols for diseases. Most of my postgraduate medical education in oncology was similar to this, with the notable exception of one mentor who strongly advocated individualized treatments. His stance was that the patient's own unique characteristics should play a major role in planning any therapy. In medical practice, this would involve extensive patient input and developing one's medical intuition to *feel* your way to determining the best therapy for the individual. I can vividly remember one patient from early in my career who would have been emotionally devastated by standard treatment but responded excellently to an individualized approach. This, and many other similar patient experiences, led me to include medical intuition in determining the best course of therapy, which resulted in a much more gratifying process and result for each patient.

One of the things Caroline does best in *The Body "Knows"* is to show us how to develop our own medical intuition. We have all had the experience of intuition—sometimes we call it a gut feeling, sometimes a hunch. But we need to enhance this skill, making it more reliable and accessible. In this book, Caroline offers specific instructions and exercises to help you reach a higher level of intuitive ability. The body is always trying to heal itself; we would not be alive for one minute if this were not the case. By using our own medical intuition, we can facilitate this process. Reading *The Body "Knows"* can connect you with your inner healer, which could have a positive, lifelong impact on your health and well-being.

— Timothy Thar, M.D., Fairfield, Iowa

Acknowledgments

I have had the privilege of knowing and working with many brilliant and courageous medical doctors, alternative health-care professionals, and practitioners, who, as mentors and friends, have helped me become who I am, and who have underscored the belief that the body *knows* what to do to get well. Each one of these people appeared at the right time to show me the next step. There are no words to express my gratitude to my all beautiful friends and family members who have supported me with their love and encouragement during the many chapters of this journey.

My thanks as well to Louise Hay and the editors and staff at Hay House, who saw my vision and helped me make it a reality.

PART I

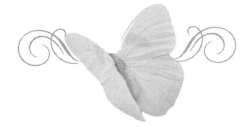

The Gift of
Medical Intuition

Chapter 1

What Is Medical Intuition?

For as long as I can remember, I've been interested in medicine. As a young child, I would run around the house in a nurse's cap, taking temperatures, checking pulses, and wrapping bandages around the imaginary wounds of my family members. When my father was studying for his final exams in tropical medicine, I'd pull a huge chair over to his desk and clamber on top of it so I could reach for the medical books that seemed twice my size. I would pore over pictures of people in the advanced stages of yaws, elephantiasis, and leprosy, trying to figure out how they got so sick. Little did I know that seeds were being planted which, decades later, would bear fruit in the exciting field of medical intuition.

Medical intuition is the ability to see beyond the normal levels of perception into the subtle levels below, pertaining to the physical body and its processes. As unusual as it may seem, many people actually have this ability. For instance, your chiropractor uses applied kinesiology, which is a form of medical intuition, to determine structural imbalances. The body *speaks* through this method, enabling the chiropractor to determine the appropriate adjustment. Applied kinesiology, or muscle testing, is now used by many alternative and mainstream health-care practitioners. It's the body's way of revealing hidden clues to the practitioner, and this system can be easily learned.

The key to medical intuition—or any other psychic or intuitive ability—is a quiet, receptive mind. A mind that is well trained in any profession will almost always develop intuitive ability. The more a person works at their craft, the more intuitive that person will become in their area of expertise. The rational or trained mind becomes the filter through which the intuitive impressions are received. Meditation, prayer, and quiet receptivity are prerequisites for this ability. Medical intuition comes from the spiritual level; it comes from God, where everything is known.

Perhaps one of the most gifted medical intuitives of our time is Caroline Myss, M.D. Her popular books *Anatomy of the Spirit* (Random House, 1997) and *Why People Don't Heal and How They Can* (Three Rivers Press, 1998) have helped thousands of people understand their illnesses from an emotional and spiritual perspective. Her stunning instincts have fascinated both lay people and professionals, and she was the one who coined the phrase *medical intuitive* to describe someone who has this gift.

Edgar Cayce is another famous medical intuitive. *There is a River: The Edgar Cayce Story,* by Thomas Sugrue (ARE Press, 1997) documents his fascinating life and abilities. This humble man practiced clairvoyant diagnosis for more than 40 years—with no medical background. He devised all of his "cures" in the sleep state or in a deep trance. People would come to him with all sorts of problems. Cayce would lie down, take a nap, or drop into this deep altered state and let the solutions for their health problems come to him. Medical doctors were constantly impressed by Cayce's level of accuracy and his specific knowledge of physical body processes, which he apparently knew nothing about when he was awake.

Belief in the person who is delivering the message and the information that is being given is a fundamental element in healing. Edgar Cayce's successes had as much to do with *the belief that people had in him* as the cures he dispensed.

My medical intuitive ability doesn't revolve around the emotional or spiritual levels or the sleep state. My eyes are wide open, I'm fully aware, and the practical suggestions drop into my mind. I always ask myself, *What does this body want?* While the emotional and spiritual levels are taken into account, my strength seems to lie specifically on the physical level, probably as a result of my training in environmental medicine, where I worked as an allergy-testing technician for many years. I will delve more deeply into my background later on in the book.

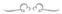

Please note that medical intuition, or any other form of alternative therapy, is never a replacement for regular medical attention. *Never give your power away or abdicate your own good judgment and common sense to any intuitive or medical practitioner.* Trust the accuracy and usefulness of the information being given to you and with your own instincts. Assess it.

Beware of medical intuitives who "see" dark masses, cancer, or other problems and offer no practical solutions. Check their references and seek a second opinion. Such an experience can be very scary. If a medical intuitive is good at what they do and are tuning in accurately, the information will *feel right to you.* When you implement the suggestions, you should feel positive results in your health. Also, always follow up with a competent medical doctor and skilled alternative practitioner in your community who can give you ongoing support. Remember that *the body only wants to repair*—we just need to give it the tools to do so.

During approximately two decades of immersion in the complementary or alternative medical field, it has been clearly revealed to me that there are certain simple principles, which when implemented can make a tremendous difference to a person's health and well-being. Think of those indigenous people who saw Columbus's ships for the first time: When their eyes were trained to see beyond their normal experience, they were open to a whole new realm of possibility.

Anyone can learn to develop intuition and increase physical body awareness—it's not the domain of a very few select people. Medical intuition, or body awareness, exists within each person. Allow yourself to hone your own instincts in ways that are appropriate and make sense to you. It takes time, practice, and a practical framework to see with a new set of eyes. There are many courses offered in medical intuition, and it's useful to learn all that you can in this regard. Although courses may be helpful, ultimately your insights will come through *you* and become defined in your own unique manner. Your instincts will develop in your own way. Trust these inclinations and utilize them for better health. In Part V of this book, I will help you develop your own gifts of intuition.

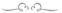

Not every body has the capacity to heal, but most people will get better—that's what the body is designed to do. Never give up on your path to wellness. If you're not yet "cured," it just means that there's something else waiting to be discovered. Optimum health is not a mystery. I have to report that people are looking all over the place for answers to their health concerns when most of the solutions are right in front of their noses. If I hadn't witnessed this dramatic transformation thousands of times in a clinical setting, I wouldn't have believed it myself. God makes things simple—

if we need something, it's never very far away. The path to wellness is like a treasure hunt—the next clue will show up when you need it, and it will lead you onward to the treasure. All of the clues, and ultimately the treasures, of optimum health are found along the way. So it is with the healing journey, which is rarely a single treatment process. Most often it's a combination of several things working together.

What we need to remember is that the body only wants to get well. It's valiantly trying to do so, every moment of our lives, at any age—we just need to give it the tools to do so. When we implement these tools, people are stunned by the level of health they can achieve.

When it comes to health, no one can deny the importance of instinct, but everyone needs to be practical. As the saying goes, "Believe in Allah but tie your camel." I'm constantly appalled by the number of people I see who don't receive appropriate medical care. Many people expect help or even miracles to come forth from alternative medical practitioners when they should be seeing a medical doctor. Take, for instance, a woman I met who obviously needed medical attention. When I asked her when she'd last seen her doctor, she replied that she hadn't consulted with a physician in more than ten years! She ended up in the hospital, and the doctor was the one who saved her. Years of resistance to a simple surgical procedure cost her big time—financially and physically.

So go to see your doctor. Get your annual checkup, blood tests, prostate-specific antigen test, rectal exam, pelvic exam, pap smear, mammogram, whatever. It's worth it. I firmly believe in having a good, working relationship with your medical doctor. You never know when he or she might be needed. Don't completely rely on your alternative practitioner. Complementary medicine means *a combination of all disciplines working together* to assist you in becoming healthy.

Remember to always get your doctor's permission before

starting any new program, and always support the medical doctors who are innovative, seeking to provide their patients with the best approaches, both complementary and traditional. We need to encourage our regular medical doctors to become knowledgeable about what we're investigating in the field of alternative health. Many traditional M.D.'s are very interested and want to learn. In the future, the most popular doctors and insurance companies will be the ones that support complementary medical disciplines.

If you're interested in environmental medicine or clinical ecology, ask your doctor to refer you to someone in your area. If you don't know where to start, call the American Holistic Medical Association (703-556-9728). The association also has a Website (**www.holisticmedicine.org**) that can direct you to appropriate services and holistically oriented medical practitioners in the United States. In Canada, contact the Canadian Complementary Medical Association at: **www.ccmadoctors.ca.**

My purpose in writing *The Body "Knows"* is to help fundamentally healthy people who suffer, as we all do from time to time, from common complaints such as gas, bloating, headaches, skin rashes, weight gain, fluid retention, poor memory, joint stiffness, sinus problems, digestive upsets, and hormonal imbalances. I felt that a simple manual, outlining the most common places to look for possible answers, would assist people in becoming more intuitive about their own bodies, thus enhancing their individual health goals.

In this book, my aim is to demystify the body's processes and create a basic foundation—a "table," if you wish—comprised of four solid legs and a sturdy top. When the table is built, a person is ready for all of the other beautiful elements of alternative health care to be placed upon it—the refinements—such as acupuncture treatments, massage therapy, chiropractic adjustments, bioresonance therapy, aroma-therapy, kinesiology, and psychotherapy.

Just give me 30 days of your life—four weeks of your time—and let's see what *your* body knows. In the next chapter, I will describe how my medical intuitive gift came to me as a result of my own health challenges.

Chapter 2

My Story

The gift of medical intuition came to me quite suddenly in the early 1980s when I was working as a physician's assistant and allergy-testing technician for a very busy medical doctor who specialized in environmental medicine. Environmental medicine deals with the human body in relationship to the environment—everything a person eats, breathes, and comes in contact with—and the effect each of these elements has on a person's body. This is the fascinating field in which I was immersed.

I'd been trained in the use of highly specialized European allergy-testing equipment. After using this equipment for about a year, I began to hear a very distinct inner voice guiding me to investigate particular areas of the body and specific substances to examine—which hadn't been ordered on the test forms. I shared the information that I was "hearing" with the physician I was working for. Fortunately, because he was a very open-minded individual, he agreed to evaluate its validity. Over the ensuing months, we arrived at a place where both of us were working as an incredible team—I intuited each patient's needs more deeply than we were able to do with the diagnostic equipment, and he used his medical knowledge in evaluation and treatment. In a very short time, because of our finely tuned results, people were getting well, and the clinic had a year-long waiting list.

This partnership continued for several years, and then I had a strong instinct to leave the clinic and open my own office. I went on to create guided-imagery audiotapes for children and adults, for which I am now rather well known. After a few years in business for myself, I was asked by a naturopathic physician to join his clinic as an allergy-testing technician. He was aware of my intuitive abilities and gratefully accepted my instinctive impressions regarding his patients. In no time, his practice was thriving.

My medical intuitive ability is very specific to the *physical* body. After nearly two decades in environmental medicine, I see the body from that perspective. To help a person, I don't have to be in their actual physical presence—in fact, all I need to know is their name and a little about them, hear their voice, or see their photograph. The minute I connect with the person seeking my help, a flood of data comes to me. The information is very specific. I can intuit foods that a person is allergic/sensitive to, perceive the main systems that may be compromised, observe the state of the gastrointestinal tract or immune system, and check for hormone imbalances or weight problems. I then look at the underlying causes of these problems, when they began, and what may have precipitated them. I also perceive suggestions regarding their diet, which supplements or botanicals they might benefit from, whether homeopathy would be helpful for them, and so on.

Other useful information is also given to me, such as the length of time for a patient's recovery, whether or not that patient will be compliant, or if indeed they are likely to recover at all. In this nearly 20-year period, I've had the privilege of being part of the assessment and treatment of more than 60,000 people.

How It All Began

I've often thought that my specific medical orientation came to me via my deceased doctor father. He died when I was 26 years old, and our relationship had never been close. In fact, it may seem strange, but I was relieved when he died. Over the years, I believe that "through the veil," or from the other side, he tried to make contact with me on a number of occasions. But, because of my feelings toward him, I pushed this connection away. Years later, after much intro-spection and deep meditative work, I accepted the nature of our relationship on a karmic level. It was necessary for the development of my potential, and I forgave him. At that moment, I was catapulted into his world—the world of medicine.

I don't feel my father's presence with me while I work, nor do I get a sense of working with specific medical guid-ance. I prefer to feel linked to the highest connection—the connection with God, or the Creator—in this endeavor. But I do believe that my father, with whom I had so much difficulty in my Earth life, is making amends from the other side.

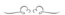

I was one of four children in a medical family. Both my father and my grandfather were physicians—my grandfather was a country doctor in the north of England, and my father was a physician with the World Health Organization and for the Ford and Rockefeller Foundations. I grew up in various countries (including Switzerland, where I attended boarding school) before returning to the West Coast and resuming my studies at a university. There I met and married my husband, and we settled down to raise our two daughters. Life was normal, easy, and predictable.

For several years, I worked as a writer for a large city newspaper and a glossy fashion magazine. My field was style and interior design—everything to do with the *outside*. Along the way, however, I became disenchanted with the preoccupation of the "plastic" exterior. How many times can you write about belts, hats, scarves, skirt lengths, and the latest fashion trends without being thoroughly bored? At that time, without knowing where to look or defining a direction, I was searching for something new. As a busy wife, mother, and freelance writer, I often termed myself a "stressed-out basket case," always trying to do too much. I sought ways to relax, and was grateful to be introduced to meditation in the early '80s—in fact, I believe that practicing meditation precipitated my ability to eventually become a medical intuitive.

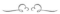

In 1983, I went for my yearly physical. I was 38 years old. I was seeing a new doctor, but there was no reason to suspect that this annual checkup would be different from any other one. I expected the usual—blood pressure check, Pap smear, a look in the ears and throat, and a few prods here and there—then I'd be given a clean bill of health for another year. But although it was difficult to put my finger on the problem, I hadn't been feeling terrific at the time—not really sick, but not really well either. I'd been having some peculiar symptoms that had me worried, such as numbness and tingling in my arms and hands, mini-blackouts, memory loss, periods of depression, and frequent states of fear and anxiety.

As I lay on the examining table, draped in a white sheet, I decided to come clean and tell this doctor everything I'd been experiencing, and risk being told it was just "battle fatigue" or "all in my head." I was reluctant to disclose my concerns—in case they might be true. After I related my worrisome signs, I went on to tell the doctor of my greatest fear. I'd been bumping into things, such as the edge of a doorway, or I'd catch my hip on a table rim or the back of a chair. I seemed to be losing my balance or my sense of perception—could all this be the dreaded warning signs of multiple sclerosis (MS)? I had a girlfriend who was afflicted with MS, and I thought that her similar early symptoms signaled the same fate for me.

After relating this bizarre history, I was expecting the usual knowing look of condescension I'd seen over the years from other doctors—silently implying that my problems were of a psychosomatic nature. Surprise! *This* doctor responded with interest and compassion and appeared to have an immediate understanding of the problem. After examining me thoroughly, she said that she suspected that allergies to certain foods and a sensitivity to yeast were the culprits. Allergies—ridiculous! Why, I'd never broken out in hives, had an asthma attack, or reacted violently to anything I'd eaten . . . I didn't think. Allergies, I concluded, were for neurotics.

The doctor waited until I had calmed down and shared how she too had suffered from similar symptoms. She suggested that a specific kind of allergist—a specialist in environmental medicine—could help. She then referred me to a doctor colleague of hers who specialized in the treatment of food allergies, the candida yeast syndrome, and environmental illness. In her opinion, it was doubtful that I had MS; more than likely, I had simple food allergies and a possible sensitivity to yeast. It was worth investigating. I look back on that day now and give thanks to this forward-thinking physician who changed the course of my life.

So, tucking the name and address of the environmental medical specialist into my purse, I wondered what the next step would be. It was November, just a few weeks before

Christmas, and no one was going to deprive me of my shortbread, eggnog, and all the other seasonal goodies that I looked forward to every year. We'd see about allergies later. I proceeded to eat and drink my way through Christmas. Then, when the last piece of chocolate had called out to be eaten, and the last crumb of Christmas cake was consumed, I was ready for my appointment.

Feeling bloated and depressed, I entered the environmental medical clinic. All of my symptoms had returned with a vengeance. How could this doctor, I thought skeptically, have an answer to such a host of problems?

The Turning Point

Clinical ecology (or environmental medicine) deals with our relationship to the environment. The approach is comprehensive and holistic. Everything a person eats, breathes, or comes into contact with can all contribute to the symptoms they may be experiencing. So, at the clinic I was referred to, a very detailed history was taken, with each complaint carefully noted. I was also asked about the foods I most often consumed, which I thought was an unusual question for a doctor to ask. I had to confess that I had frequent cravings for sweets and breads.

The next day, during several hours of testing, I was to learn more about the effects of food and chemicals on the body. The kind of testing I was subjected to is called intradermal testing, and it involves the injection of a concentrated amount of each allergen or substance under the skin, at ten-minute intervals. The patient's pulse rate is taken, reactions noted, and a wheal or bump at the injection site is measured. After ten minutes, each test is "neutralized," and individuals are brought back to normal so that subsequent tests can continue. The substance being tested isn't revealed to the patient until that test is completed. In this testing area,

I was fascinated to see ten different people react in many different ways to foods found in the typical shopping cart. We discussed their reactions:

- Bill, a robust but slightly overweight 35-year-old, was experiencing a runny nose, streaming eyes, and a red face from apples—one of his favorite foods. An hour later, when tested for wheat, he fell fast asleep.

- Arlene, an attractive 30-year-old executive, had suffered from depression all her life. She started crying uncontrollably in the middle of a conversation. What could cause such a reaction? Eggs. She loved them, ate two for breakfast, and would even whip up an omelette for a late-night snack.

- Arran, a boisterous nine-year-old, jumped up and down in a hyperactive and aggressive fashion in reaction to sugar, beef, and milk. Ten minutes later, a neutralizing dose of the same allergen cleared his symptoms and returned him to a calm and agreeable state.

It seemed that all of us in that testing room reacted to the foods that we ate most frequently or to which we were addicted. Wheat, dairy products, and corn appeared to be the worst offenders. The phrase "You are what you eat" took on new meaning for us.

In my case, milk brought on stomach cramps, postnasal drip, and a dry cough—obviously the "healthy" cottage cheese salad that I ate every day for lunch was doing me no good. Wheat induced a fuzzy head and exhaustion; I could hardly keep my eyes open during the test. I was sad to think that I'd have to give up making the eight loaves of bread that graced the family table each week. Bread was supposed to be the staff of life, but if I kept eating it, it would take more than a staff to prop me up!

The testing continued. Oranges gave me a pounding sinus headache and pulsating temples. What would I do without my morning O.J.? I experienced fatigue; and pain in my hands, and a raised pulse when exposed to chicken. Potatoes caused fatigue, pain in my wrists, hands, and knees. One by one, the basic foods were being crossed off my list—what was I going to eat? Coffee elicited exhaustion; I knew that caffeine made me hyper, but the bean itself made me tired. Corn gave me a headache, stomachache, and a spacey feeling. Corn? Why, I rarely ate corn except fresh from the farmers' market in the summer. But it turns out that corn is everywhere—most packaged and canned products contain corn, and even baby powder and some toothpastes do. It's not so easy to eliminate.

I was then tested for common inhalants—the things that we breathe in the environment. This, too, was very revealing. Chlorine caused fatigue and pulsating temples—even the tap water had to go! Formaldehyde brought on a headache and that foggy feeling again, as well as exhaustion and an increased pulse rate. Formaldehyde is impregnated into synthetic fibers. This was an important link for me because I always felt tired and developed a mild headache when I was researching clothing stores for my weekly fashion column. Many women told me that they found shopping draining. Could it be that the clothing selection was not as overwhelming as the fumes?

Surely the tests were finished. At this point, my very lifestyle and career was being challenged. It was hard to accept all of this information at once. But then they brought out one more test—for a yeast extract called candida albicans. This experiment took 30 minutes.

Within ten minutes of this test, I had a dry cough and felt that old familiar sensation of panic and anxiety across my chest. A few minutes later, this turned into depression. Then my neck and shoulders became stiff, and the numbness and tingling in my arms and hands became severe. At last, all that I needed to know was revealed to me in black and white. I almost cried with relief that here, finally, was an answer. These reactions indicated that my "wholesome" diet and candida yeast were at the root of my physical symptoms.

After the testing was complete, I crawled home with a terrible headache. The decision was clear—I had to temporarily eliminate my favorite foods so that my body could rest from their toxic effects, and I needed to take medication to eradicate the candida albicans yeast strain.

Within three weeks of taking a specific substance to stamp out the candida yeast, and making the necessary dietary changes, I began to feel better. The pain in my neck and shoulders, and the tingling down my arms, had diminished. I knew I had made a breakthrough when I was backing the car out of the driveway and I could turn my head without pain. I adhered very closely to my new dietary restrictions for several months—which was no mean feat, and added considerable stress to my busy lifestyle as a mother and newspaper columnist.

But my energy returned. I was no longer tired and worn out, and the great bonus was that I could eat as much as I wanted as long as I stayed away from *offending foods*. And, I *lost* weight. Most days I felt like a 21-year-old. My skin cleared up, and my brain and memory returned to normal clarity. My temperament and attitude toward life was one of joyous anticipation. This is how we're all supposed to feel!

All my symptoms had disappeared, never to return. I was a convert. I dragged my family, all my friends, and anyone who would listen to see the allergist. I was charged with vitality and made the inner commitment that I was ready for a new direction. I didn't have to wait long.

My disenchantment with newspaper writing and the world of fashion was the signal for life to open a different door for me.

After several months of being his patient, the allergist approached me and asked me to join his clinic. He realized that I had good communication skills, was compliant on the new program, had a medical background, and was keenly interested in the whole field of environmental medicine—so he asked me to become trained as his assistant and allergy-testing technician. I was delighted.

This involved an intense, year-long, total immersion program with much studying, training, and attendance at seminars. I even got to go on a trip to England to observe brilliant, cutting-edge medical doctors, who were among the most respected in their field, doing similar, more advanced work. I was in total joy—I had found my life's purpose.

Chapter 3

Breaking Through
and Seeing Beyond

In the early 1980s, the terms *environmental medicine* and *clinical ecology* weren't widely known. At the clinic, we attracted patients who had been chronically ill for many years and had been around the block and then some trying to get help. It was very revealing to me that in a matter of just a few months, sometimes even weeks, people who had been offered no hope elsewhere were finding that their symptoms were being relieved. It didn't seem to matter what age they were. Even a person in their 70s or 80s could make a dramatic health turnaround if they were given the information and tools they needed to effect positive change. We were also able to help children with behavior or learning problems, allergies, and many other specialized complaints.

The usual chronic problems for adults were headaches, fatigue, weight problems, joint aches, and allergies, just to name a few. Because I'd been a writer and reporter, I naturally began to ask the patients questions such as, "When were you last well?" Invariably the person would answer, "I was fine up until my mother died," or "Everything was great until my marriage broke up," or "Before I lost my job." There always seemed to be an emotional component to their illness, even though the progression of their condition may have been subtle or undefined.

Like most places that test for and treat allergies, we utilized intradermal (under the skin) and sublingual (under the tongue) tests to determine allergies and sensitivities. But we also used various innovative approaches in the clinic, which for that time were quite advanced but are now widely used in environmental medicine clinics in North America and Europe. One of these progressive methods involved the use of phenolics, which are core chemical elements, or aromatic compounds, found in foods, vitamins, minerals, hormones, and neurotransmitters. If a person is sensitive to a certain food—perhaps a grain such as wheat (flour)—they can be neutralized for the aromatic compound or the phenolic chemical that's found in that particular grain family. This neutralizes, or takes away, the adverse effect that person may experience when exposed to the wheat or any other substance containing that core phenolic element. Along with avoiding the food itself for a limited period of time, phenolic neutralization seemed to be very effective. Even people with hormone imbalances could be neutralized for the core component of an appropriate hormone, thereby improving hormonal functions.

It was fascinating to witness dramatic improvements in people as they were neutralized for these substances. I would marvel at these transformations day after day. We were also able to neutralize people for colds and flu—many times our whole treatment area was filled up with people in various stages of a flu or cold. We took them through the illness by degrees, giving them neutralizing drops of the viruses themselves, which were placed under their tongues.

During this very intense period, I had the privilege of working with several of the finest doctors in the field of environmental medicine, whose courage and bravery I want to fully acknowledge in these pages. I was also privy to cutting-edge material and treatments that these doctors were researching. In addition, there was a select support network of other professionals to whom our patients were referred for acupuncture, chiropractic, massage, hair analysis, holistic dentistry, chelation therapy, kinesiology, and counseling. This was complementary medicine at its best.

The bulk of our clinical work centered around the identification of allergies or sensitivities to common foods, inhalants and environmental factors, and the treatment of the candida yeast syndrome or chronic candidiasis. It seemed that nearly every person who visited our clinic was riddled with this yeast. It was easy to treat, and when it was eradicated, each person's energy returned, almost as if by magic. People were given a chance to experience total health—for the first time.

The Diagnostics

The term *allergy* refers to a severe reaction to a substance, which results in what is called *anaphylactic shock*. At that point, the patient may need to be rushed to an emergency room or be given a shot of adrenaline to counteract the effects of the allergen in question. Bee stings, spider bites, nuts, certain fruits, shellfish, and various other substances can cause this reaction in some people. In this book, I'm referring to *sensitivities*, particularly in food. Sensitivities imply that there's a delayed, subtle, or unidentified reaction with no known cause—to food or any other substance. In this case, a patient may experience headaches, digestive problems, or skin rashes, which although uncomfortable in nature, don't require emergency medical attention; therefore, they're not considered to be true allergies. I'll use the two terms synonymously.

My role as an allergy-testing technician involved the use of very sensitive, electro-diagnostic equipment, which was a difficult system to learn, but I seemed to have a knack for it. This type of testing meant that we were able to determine—in a very rapid and painless manner—food allergies and sensitivities; organ, hormone, and neurotransmitter imbalances; vitamin and mineral deficiencies; pollen, inhalant, and mold allergies; chemical sensitivities; metal toxicity; and body toxins.

The principle behind electro-diagnostic testing is that all things have a resonating frequency—the human body, plants, animals, foods, chemicals, and everything found in nature. These materials oscillate or vibrate at a certain frequency (which I will discuss in Chapter 14). This theory is based on quantum physics and is aptly described by Gary Zukav, Ph.D., in his book *The Dancing Wu Li Masters* (Bantam, 1994).

From this type of testing, we can determine if the samples, allergens, or individual substances are vibrating at the same frequency, or are in harmony with the patient or not. The patient holds a part of the equipment, and the allergy tester uses a probe to touch a designated acupuncture point on the patient's finger. Then each testing vial or sample is placed near the patient, and depending on several indicators, a positive or negative response is determined.

Most people prefer this form of testing over the sublingual or intradermal testing, which is laborious, expensive, painful, and potentially reactive. The electro-diagnostic method is also great for kids—no pain! In less than half an hour, the patient is given a thorough and complete workup, and their results are available immediately.

Because we saw so many patients in the clinic—about 50 a day, and I performed about 200 tests on each person—I became very intuitive about my testing. The equipment became an extension of me. When I picked up a testing vial or sample, I would feel a positive or negative response in my own body. The intuitive process was beginning to unfold.

A Life-Changing Event

One morning, I arrived at the clinic early. I needed to prepare some of the neutralizing drops that we'd be using for the day's patients. As I was working quietly at my desk, I noticed a bright light begin to form on the back wall of the testing room. As it began to get brighter, I felt intense heat in my own body. Suddenly, in the center of this expanded, blinding white light, the rarefied outline of a figure appeared—a presence, a radiant being, a messenger . . . an angel.

I stared, awestruck, as this presence spoke to me, not with words that I could hear out loud, but words that I could hear *within* me. "Behold the Angel. Will you do my work?" was what I heard. The effect of this presence seemed to pierce right through me to the core of my being. I sat and gazed in wonder. I wasn't afraid. It was as if I had met this presence before, and it had traveled with me throughout my life. Without words, I acknowledged that I would do "the work"—whatever it was—and in an instant, the vision disappeared.

I couldn't believe what had happened. Time stood still—what seemed like an eternity was actually a wink of an eye. I wanted to pinch myself to know that what I'd seen was real. I was in a state of euphoria and floated around the office like a puppet on a string. As I wandered around, completely elated, I was filled with the presence of love and inner knowing. Suddenly, I was attracted to a huge bouquet of flowers on the reception desk. I put my ear to the flowers and could hear tiny reedlike notes emanating from them, which I later discovered was the "music of the spheres." That particular day gave me the opportunity to experience the deeper meaning of life on all levels, and to understand why we're put on this Earth.

When someone has been touched deeply by the presence of the Holy Spirit, a cornucopia of gifts is given to them. This could be the capacity to heal, the capability to hear God's voice (or the small, still voice within), the proficiency to *know* and understand at the very deepest levels, and the ability to experience an abundance of creativity. When a person has the presence of the Holy Spirit within them, they become an instrument, divinely inspired. This peak, spiritual experience came to me suddenly—one moment I didn't have the ability of insight, the next moment I did. I believe that my willingness and desire to become an instrument for good in the world precipitated these events.

—⟨⟩⟨⟩—

As soon as the patients arrived at the clinic that day, I could see the auras, or electromagnetic fields, around them. And I seemed to know on a deeper level why they were coming to the clinic, what they had to tell me, and what I had to share with them. This was a powerful, compelling experience for which I wasn't fully prepared, and it heralded an infusion of the gifts of the spirit, which were to be bestowed upon me.

From then on, all I had to do was see a patient's name on the chart and I would immediately receive a flood of information about their treatment—which compounds to use, exactly where to start each treatment remedy, or anything else that was important to know. Fortunately, I had developed a comfortable rapport with the doctor, and as soon as I was able, I discussed the information I was being given with him. I will be forever grateful that he was open-minded and allowed me to communicate any of the impressions I experienced regarding his patients, and he was willing to incorporate this knowledge into his practice.

It took about two years for my instinct to become integrated so that it didn't overwhelm me. At first, I couldn't turn the ability off—I was tuning in to bodies day and night. But eventually things settled down, and it just became a normal, everyday part of my life. I was lucky to have excellent support and spiritual mentoring during this time, which helped me understand and live with the wonderful gift that had fallen into my lap.

From those intense, early beginnings, my work as a medical intuitive has become more refined. Although I no longer use the diagnostic equipment on a daily basis, it's as if I have the equipment with me when I work with patients or clients. I see the body from that perspective. Every test vial that I have ever used clicks through my mind, assisting me in the identification of certain imbalances and body processes.

Pondering the Meaning

It took some time to ponder the significance of that experience in my office. What was the meaning of "Will you do my work?" My first thought was that there must be some very special work for me to do, or, could it be that the work I needed to do was on *myself?*

I immediately set out to become a more loving presence in my own life. This was a transformational concept, as I instantly became conscious and present in every single interaction, every moment of the day. I knew that each person in the clinic would be the test of this commitment. They could be frustrated, irritable, weary, and lacking in hope, and I had to see beyond their outer behavior and recognize that they were precious souls traveling on the same path that I was. My role was to be present and loving, and to visualize them healthy and well.

I practiced this new state of being in my own family, especially with my children, who were teenagers at the time. There's nothing more challenging than seeing a teenager as a *person,* apart from their rather baffling adolescent behavior. I tried to see my daughters for the radiant beings that they were, and for the wise and beautiful women that they were becoming. I ignored their negative behaviors, and more often than not, they showed me the positive side of themselves. I showered them with love and validation, which has had a tremendous beneficial effect to this day. I feel lucky to have had a wake-up call about how to truly interact with people on these deep and meaningful levels.

From that pivotal morning on, things became very accelerated in the clinic. We were able to bypass some of the slow, laborious treatments and simplify our approaches, because the doctor himself was becoming more intuitive. We used to get together for a couple of hours on the weekends to intuit protocols and new techniques. What a team we were!

My skill in allergy testing and intuition increased. I would hear a distinct voice guiding me to items that didn't even appear on the test forms. I would be directed to tell the doctor that a particular patient might benefit from a certain injectable vitamin or some other form of therapy. Sometimes it was combinations of phenolic compounds and other substances that we routinely used in treatment. I could pick up a bottle of vitamins or some other substance and *know* whether it would be effective for the patient, and what the dosage would be and how long the substance was required to be taken.

It was extremely fulfilling work, and these were high times. But I was also getting exhausted. The clinic opened early, and we would see countless people every day, month after month, with no relief in sight. I was getting intuitive nudges that soon it would be time to leave the clinic, which made me sad, but I also realized that it had to be done.

The next step was revealed to me in a powerful dream shortly after I left the clinic. For the previous three years, along with everything else that I was doing, I'd been studying relaxation therapy. God knows I needed to relax! I discovered that I had a talent for creating individual, guided-imagery audiotapes, which helped adults and children to relax, sleep better, and feel more positive about life. So, one morning, I awoke from a very graphic dream that showed me a complete set of audiotapes designed to help children feel positive and loved—which is the basis of good health! I was also shown in the dream that these audiotapes would be teamed with a cuddly doll in the shape of an angel. At last, it was time to further understand the meaning of "Will you do my work?"

I opened a small office, and many people asked to have individualized audiotapes created for their own needs. Many of my clients were children who had a variety of ailments and concerns such as head injuries, burns, amputations, divorce, abuse, sleeplessness, and the aftereffects of cancer treatments. It was always a pleasure to create audiotapes for these kids, and I felt that the words on the tapes were spiritually inspired. I called them *Sleep Talking*® tapes. (For more information on my products, please see page 297.)

Although I'd started working on audiotape and angel doll products (which to date have helped countless children around the world), I was never very far away from the medicine. After several years of relaxation therapy work, I was drawn back into the medical world. I was asked by a naturopathic physician and his wife (also a naturopath) to join their clinic as an allergy-testing technician on a part-time basis. I was thrilled to be back in a clinical setting, and this doctor also knew of my intuitive abilities and welcomed the information that I received about his patients. It never ceased to amaze us both that my "test" results were constantly validated by a patient's history. I would pick up on an imbalance, and sure enough, it would be there on the chart.

While I was at this clinic, I had the chance to witness some of the eclectic treatment modalities offered by naturopathic physicians, and to see the benefits of injectable and intravenous vitamins. We would often see patients with severe chronic illness—chronic fatigue syndrome (CFS), cancer, or other serious conditions—who benefited tremendously from these injections. The aim of injectable supplementation is to transport the nutrients into the bloodstream—fast. This is another important modality that patients can explore, especially if they're recovering from an acute infection or battling a serious illness.

Going My Own Way

Eventually I felt compelled to forge my own path with my medical intuitive ability. At first, I resisted it, feeling that it was only appropriate to be used in a professional medical setting. After all, I had grown up in a medical family, and I was raised with the notion that only the doctor has the power to cure disease. But I could never resist the desire to help when it was needed: I jotted down programs for people on napkins in restaurants, or made a suggestion in passing when it was required. It just evolved—and people all over the world started to contact me.

To me, medical intuition is a very simple, natural, and straightforward ability that anyone can learn. I tend to always see the body in a state of wellness. I don't dwell on what's negative or out of balance; rather, I focus on what might be helpful to correct the situation.

As I've previously mentioned, I don't need to be in the physical presence of the person who seeks my help. I can look at a photo, hear a name, or tune in to someone as they speak to me on the telephone. From the sound of their voice, I seem to pick up any allergies or sensitivities they have to common foods, detect the presence of the yeast syndrome (which I perceive as a sweet, sickly odor), as well as determine any environmental factors that may be affecting them. I consider my work to be a basic introduction to the healing journey.

When I'm not working, I "practice" what I do by "scoping out" or "reading" people as they walk past me while I take my daily two-mile walks along the ocean. There's always a feeling of sadness within me when I see an overweight person lumbering past, huffing, puffing, and sweating. I would just love to be able to come right out and say, "Just avoid dairy products and you'll lose all that weight."

I can "see through" people and *know* that they don't need to be sick. It's a challenge *not* to look at times—such as when I see a mother reaching for the container of milk while her child sits in the shopping cart with red, puffy eyes, an obvious sign of an allergic reaction. I've cut my teeth, in a medical intuitive sense, by "scoping out" entire movie theaters. On many occasions, I'd check each person, row by row, for allergies and organ system imbalances. This formed the beginning of my group intuitive assessment process, which I currently use in all the cities that I visit. During this procedure, I tune in to each person and arrange the people in groups according to their possible needs and potential imbalances.

In the next chapter, I'll show you how your physical body and personality fit into four key body systems, and how imbalances in these areas can lead to ill health.

PART II

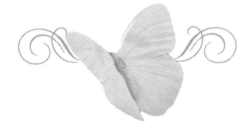

The Body Knows

Chapter 4

Recognizing Key Body Systems

When I look at a body, I immediately get a sense of which systems are "down" or in need of correction. When I was an allergy-testing technician, the first test panel I performed on each patient was called a "pretest," which enabled the doctors to determine the key systems that were out of balance. Thanks to thousands of patients and years of testing this particular panel, I am now able to determine system stress quite naturally.

After many years as a medical intuitive, I began to see patterns in people, as well as certain characteristic profiles that seemed to be identifiable. This chapter will help you understand the systems in your own body that may be stressed, and show you how to identify useful methods of correction.

The Different Body Types

The central nervous system, for example, involves any affliction related to nerves: tension, agitation, overreaction, lack of calmness, premature aging, mood swings, shakiness, heart palpitations, adrenal stress, or the inability to handle sugars and stimulants. The digestive system involves problems in the stomach, the small and large intestine and bowels; weight issues; food allergies; poor absorption; sugar and fat handling; and any other aspect of digestion.

Each system that's out of balance can be tracked or monitored to show how an imbalance might impact the entire body. When a system is corrected, many other related processes in the body have the capacity to remedy themselves. From my intuitive perspective, I see most people falling into four distinct categories. I intuitively assess all these people in terms of the body systems that are out of balance.

1. The body system that's out of whack for most people is the central nervous system. So I call this body type **CNS**, for Central Nervous System stress.

2. I named the second most common group **DLH**—for Digestive, Lymphatic, Hormonal stress—due to this type's particular unbalanced systems.

3. Occasionally, I do see people who have a combination of CNS and DLH stresses. I call these people **The Others.**

4. I've termed the rare people I see who are complicated or seriously ill **The Tricky People.**

The Central Nervous System (CNS) Type

This is the type of person I see most often. These people are what I call "short-wired" or on the ragged edge. On an energetic level, I see their nerves like the insulation on telephone wires, which over time have become stripped and broken in places, exposing the delicate wires underneath to the elements. If you think of a boat, a CNS person's profile would resemble the sail—catching the wind and moving the boat forward. CNS people often experience great emotional hills and valleys, and characteristically give their power away or give credence to elements outside of themselves. They're often very future oriented—rarely do they take the time to stop and enjoy the moment or smell the flowers, since their minds are projected ahead to the next task. CNS types believe that it's all up to them—they're the "doers" of this world. "I can do it myself," they'll often say. They are usually very intense, bright, energetic, pleaser types, all too often saying yes to things they don't really want to do. At times they can be on the edge of burnout and tend to have two distinct modes of behavior—one is full-steam ahead, and the other is full stop!

CNS types are quite often slender and wiry, but they're just as likely to have weight problems. These people tend to age early in life, and their skin can wrinkle prematurely because of their intense nature and frequent lack of fats and oils. They may have rashes and skin problems, and can suffer from brittle bones, due to their poor absorption of nutrition. They may also have very *driven* personalities and often have stressed adrenal glands or hormone imbalances. I've noticed that almost all light-haired people are CNS types.

On a higher, more spiritual level, the key word for a CNS person is *trust.* I suspect that these people were given very little validation as young children, and therefore have found their place in the world by producing, pleasing, doing, and giving to others. By constantly doing for others, a CNS person ensures that no one will ever do anything for themselves. They're often disappointed in relationships, as their need for nurturing is frequently overridden by their desire to keep the peace and make things right with their partners. About 70 percent of the people I see are CNS types.

Common imbalances in CNS people include: sleep problems, sugar-handling issues, digestive disorders, hyperimmunity (an overreactive immune system), hormone imbalances, urinary tract problems, memory loss, adrenal exhaustion, poor absorption, and brittle bones. Chemicals in the environment—such as air pollution, tobacco smoke, chemicals and perfumes—can also adversely affect these individuals.

Are you a CNS (central nervous system) type? Please answer the following questions:

- Do you consume caffeine and other stimulants?

- Do stimulants make you nervous?

- Do you have cravings for sweets?

- When you eat sweets or starches/carbohydrates by themselves, do you feel more edgy or nervous afterward?

- Are you spacey or light-headed if you don't eat on time?

- Do you get urinary tract infections?

- Do you have difficulty digesting certain foods?

- Are your nails brittle or do they break easily?

- Is your hair limp and dry?

- Are you confident, or do you give your power away to others?

- Do you drive yourself beyond your physical limits?

If you answered yes to many of these questions, you're a CNS type. Read on for some helpful hints to deal with central nervous system stresses.

Useful Solutions for CNS Types

- *Remove stimulants*—Because you have a tendency toward *burnout*, the first thing you should eliminate is all stimulants. I suggest that CNS types take a two-week break from caffeine, refined sugar, and chocolate. Then, as an experiment, add these items back into your diet and see how wired and frazzled you feel. Obviously, you should avoid cigarettes, alcohol, and recreational drugs. You're so sensitive that each of these stimulants will have an immediate effect on your entire system—often negatively.

  For example, if you're a CNS stress person with a headache, you'd take a pain reliever and would be assured that the medicine will work for you very quickly. The same principle applies to a cup of coffee, a chocolate bar, or an alcoholic beverage. You're wired in such a way that even a small amount of a stimulant can so alter you chemically that you'll be rendered angry, irrational, emotional, or unbalanced in the process.

- *Calm and soothe*—Your main focus is to *calm down*. You're usually very expressive emotionally—you'll cry, wail, and let everyone know that you're having a bad day or other painful experience. You're not afraid to show your emotions, either positively or negatively. Meditation, contemplation, being in nature, and anything to do with water will help calm you. Soothing music, walking by a lake or the sea, the sound of ocean waves on the stereo at home, soaking in soothing baths, rocking in a chair, cuddling, and pampering will all help to rebuild the CNS profile.

- *Balance body chemistry with nutrition, foods, and supplementation*—Most CNS types have sugar-handling problems. Many of you are hypoglycemic or borderline diabetic. You need to be aware of your need for *protein.* Unless a starchy, carbohydrate snack is combined with protein, you'll most likely feel off-kilter, tired, spacey, light-headed, or irritable within about a half hour. Even a muffin or bagel consumed at the wrong time by a CNS type will convert very quickly to sugar. Therefore, you'll feel much more balanced with the addition of protein in your diet at every meal and snack.

  The protein can come in any form to which you're not allergic. Nuts, seeds, and nut butters can be good snacks. The frequent consumption of eggs, chicken, turkey, fish, beans, soy, and red meats—along with liberal amounts of vegetables, nonallergic starches, and healthy fats such as essential fatty acids, olive oil, or butter—can assist you in feeling harmonious on the physical level. You may also want to talk to your doctor about supplementation for your adrenal glands.

- *Improve digestion and absorption*—The most common emotional trait in a CNS person is *giving power away*—that is, giving credence to, or dwelling on, past issues, people, places, and things that are outside of you. You constantly look to others to make you happy. You experience this loss of energy or confidence through your stomach and intestinal area—your "guts." Working on confidence, assertiveness, and staying in your power will be a lifelong process for you.

  Often you'll have poor digestion and elimination, and therefore poor assimilation or utilization of the foods you're eating. You often have stop-and-start bowel movements. Intuitively, when I look at the intestinal tract of a typical CNS type, I can usually see that the person is not soaking up the nutrients from their food, and that the mechanics for absorbing these nutrients may be depleted. This is particularly true of an elderly person. If the body isn't absorbing nutrition, cells aren't being adequately rebuilt, calcium isn't being taken into bones, and nutrients aren't being transported to calm and repair nerves. Because of a sensitive digestive tract, a CNS person will often have allergies to common foods, which can trigger gut reactions. Therefore, the use of specific digestive enzymes can be beneficial in increasing absorption levels.

- *Choose supplements to repair stressed nerves*—As a CNS person, you'll want to take full advantage of the nighttime sleep cycle for the absorption of certain nutrients, particularly calcium. When taken at bedtime, calcium accompanied by certain supplemental oils can soothe the brain and coat the nerves while you sleep. Many times I will intuitively sense that a bedtime toddy, made up of calcium, nutritional oils, and soothing teas can help send you off to dreamland—as well as restore ragged nerve endings.

- *Remember who you are*—Anyone who wants to get a job done should call upon a CNS person. You're usually driven, reliable, results oriented, and will go the extra mile—often at your own expense. However, you need lots of nurturing, validation, and support, but you get very little of it, often because you're such a giver and doer. You usually put yourself last and often have difficulty taking care of your own needs. You rarely give yourself love, validation, and encouragement. Look at yourself in the mirror, and tell yourself how valuable and precious you are, and how you deserve rest and nurturing. As you drift off to sleep, tell yourself you're special, loved, and needed in the world.

The Digestive, Lymphatic, Hormonal (DLH) Type

If CNS types are the sails in the boat, then DLH types are the anchors, meaning that these people are usually steady and rock solid. As opposed to the CNS type, the DLH type usually keeps their emotions well hidden, and will only reveal their true emotional nature if pressed, or when they feel it's very safe to do so. These are the slow and silent types, working behind the scenes, willing to be the "wind beneath the wings" of the CNS types, who are more likely to want to shine in the spotlight. A great marriage or partnership would be created between a CNS person and a DLH type.

A DLH type will commonly manifest food allergies, fluid retention, hormone imbalances, lymphatic problems, cardiac and circulatory problems, and assorted processes and blockages that I see energetically as *hardening* or *knots* of one sort or another within any of their systems. Often these people can have high cholesterol or heart problems. Endocrine imbalances, weight problems, dark circles under the eyes, acne, oily skin, and low thyroid function often show up in this type of person. They can also have a tendency toward constipation and poorly functioning livers. The DLH type has trouble letting go. They can harbor resentments, and because they often keep emotions buried, their anger can be a slow burn just below the surface—whereas the CNS types are ready to express their irritability and frustration if life throws them a curve and they're chemically and nutritionally unable to handle it.

I often find that dark-haired people are DLH types, often of ethnic origin. Hispanics, African Americans, Native Americans, and some olive-skinned European cultures frequently show up in the DLH category. These people usually display a certain depth, heaviness, or sense of calmness or control. About 30 percent of the people I see have issues with the digestive, lymphatic, and hormonal systems.

Are you a DLH (digestive, lymphatic, hormonal) type? Please answer the following questions:

- Do you feel like a solid, steady sort of person?

- Are you prone to gaining weight?

- Do you have a tendency to manufacture lumps, bumps, or cysts?

- Do you feel full or bloated after meals?

- Is your face puffy?

- Are your sinuses congested?

- Is your energy sluggish?

- Is it difficult to get moving at times?

- Do you have difficulty expressing your emotions?

- Do you hold on to anger and resentment?

- Is your anger a slow burn or deeply buried?

- Is your sex drive low?

If you answered yes to many of these questions, you're a DLH type. Read on for some helpful hints to deal with digestive, lymphatic, hormonal stresses.

Useful Solutions for DLH Types

- *Identify food allergies and factors in fluid retention*—Typically, you'll have allergies to common foods—usually dairy products. Most forms of cow's milk (except for butter, which contains very few milk solids) can cause digestive upsets, sinus congestion, and fluid retention.

For some, dairy can contribute to lymphatic blockages and the production of lumps and cysts beneath the skin. It can be helpful to institute a period of avoidance from dairy products. This takes the pressure off the digestive, lymphatic, and immune systems. You should be aware of any other food sensitivity you may have, and make sure that you're having a normal bowel movement each day.

- *Exercise*—DLH types need to exercise on a regular basis. Because of your tendency to be stuck emotionally, activity and movement will help "unglue" you. Lymph drainage massage and bodywork can get things moving. Put on some lively music and dance. Good-quality sex can also be very useful. When I see DLH types, I'd like to roll you around in the mud— loosen you up a little.

- *Watch your hormone balance*—The DLH type can be prone to hormone imbalances. Males often show up with depleted energy, decreased libido, and low testosterone levels. Both males and females almost always have low, or borderline-low, thyroid function. Specific balancing of the endocrine system can help increase energy and stamina and get your engines revved up for improved metabolism and weight reduction.

- *Move forward in life*—On a higher or spiritual level, the key phrase for a DLH type is *letting go*—letting go of past resentment, grievances, and anger—often toward yourself for missed opportunities, or for those occasions when you wanted to step into the ring but were afraid to do so. You can have deeply buried, slowly boiling anger. As opposed to a CNS type whose anger is much quicker to spark, DLH types need positive outlets for their anger, such as movement and exercise. Because you have a huge capacity to love, tolerate, and embrace, you often have unmet emotional needs. It will take someone special to penetrate the deeper reaches of your soul, and to unlock the emotions that you can keep well hidden.

The Others

The Others are combinations of the first two types. They may be predominately CNS, but will have a little DLH thrown in, or vice versa. Often, as I see these people on an energetic level, they will have processes and systems that are complicated, knotted up, or hardened.

When I look at any physical body, I see it like a river, which has the possibility of flowing smoothly, providing that certain elements are in place. The Others are the people who may have boulders, sticks, and logjams in their rivers, and sometimes it can be questionable as to whether they will unblock or not. Often people in this category are medicated or overmedicated.

On an emotional level, they may have experienced traumas and severe emotional upheavals. It's not that these people are beyond hope, but in some cases, it will take a number of skilled practitioners working together to help them. The key concepts for The Others are mobilizing the *will to live,* taking a good look at the elements of health, embracing many options, and moving back into the mainstream of life. The Others make up a small percentage of the people who come to me for help.

The Tricky People

Thankfully, very few people I see are The Tricky People. These individuals usually have serious illnesses or diseases, chronic environmental problems, physical disabilities, and complex problems that are far beyond my ken.

An angel, least of all me, would fear to tread in their midst to help them.

Many of these people have been extremely dedicated to their healing processes, have consulted with health-care professionals of all kinds, have spent thousands of dollars trying to get well, and still remain ill. Some of them have been sick, immobilized, or confined to wheelchairs all of their lives. As I meet them, I'm always thankful for the level of health I enjoy. Not that many years ago, I too became close to being one of The Tricky People.

I look at each person individually and assess whether I might have a useful nugget or a pearl to offer. I do my best to refer these people to a good local practitioner who can assist them on an ongoing basis. I always encourage them and offer them hope. The body knows what to do. Even Tricky People can turn around. I know. I've seen it.

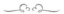

As you're reading about body profiles, remember that *every body is different.* Even though people may be similar types and share common traits, there are no blanket solutions. "What does this body want?" is the question we need to ask.

Popular books and information—which suggest that everyone should take this or that herb or supplement or follow a certain plan—fall short, because of their lack of understanding regarding the uniqueness of the individual. *The body knows.* My days in the clinic gave me a graphic education in this important truth.

In the next chapter, I'll introduce you to the cornerstone of my medical intuitive work, where on a practical level, I believe that you'll see the quickest and most dramatic benefits with respect to your energy and health. We're going to delve into the fascinating realm of the effect that some foods have on the body, and we'll also look at a seemingly innocent little yeast that may actually be making you sick.

Chapter 5

Candida Yeast and Food Allergies

Now that you've identified your body's system profile and have noted methods for improvement in that area, the next step is to act as an intuitive detective. For instance, learning about candida albicans yeast, as well as common food allergies, could give you important clues to the state of your health.

What Is Candida Albicans Yeast?

The eradication of candida albicans yeast should be the cornerstone in your desire for optimum health. This strain of yeast—which occurs naturally in the digestive tract, skin, mouth, and nose—is present in the mucous membranes of all human beings. In a healthy state, candida albicans, other yeasts, and fungi exist in balance with normal intestinal flora, which is necessary for digestion, assimilation of nutrition, and the prevention of infection. But under certain conditions, this yeast can increase rapidly, and in its fungal form, can overgrow the normal, beneficial bacteria. Due to the overuse of antibiotics, increased use of birth control pills, and poor diets, many people's normal intestinal flora becomes imbalanced, and this ubiquitous, ever-present yeast proliferates. Cravings for sweets and starches intensify the situation.

Candida is just as timely and important now as it was in the mid-1980s, when William Crook, a medical doctor from Tennessee, wrote *The Yeast Connection Handbook* (Professional Books, 1999). Dr. Crook is well known for his mainstream research and documentation in the area of candidiasis (the syndrome caused by an overgrowth of candida), and has written many books on the subject.

Dr. Crook expanded the groundbreaking work of another doctor, Orian Truss, whose book *The Missing Diagnosis* (**www.missingdiagnosis.com**) identified candida yeast and its links to many diseases. When I first read *The Missing Diagnosis*, I was stunned when I read the case histories, particularly those concerning women. I nearly cried when I read how similar their symptoms were to my own and to many of the women that we treated in a clinical setting. Now there are many popular books available on the subject, and yeast-eradication kits and supplements are readily available in health-food stores.

Over many years, I've seen the benefit of treating yeast in almost every single patient, and I've observed that this condition is almost always correctable. Candida albicans yeast can affect either sex at any age, including infancy. It appears to be more prevalent in women—probably due to the nature of their delicate endocrine systems—but many men suffer from it as well. In adults, this syndrome (and its inherent imbalances), is almost always diagnosed as a mental problem. The patient is usually told that it's "all in your head" and is referred for psychotherapy. But the rapid disappearance of all symptoms when the yeast is treated illustrates the capacity of this fungus to be part of many serious imbalances.

Because candida albicans is fed on starches and sugars,

it rapidly proliferates. An overgrowth of candidiasis can and does recur. Two common symptoms associated with candida are fatigue and sugar cravings. Once the overgrowth of candida is under control, these sugar cravings diminish. Candida can cause a myriad of symptoms such as gas, bloating, weight gain, digestive disorders, headaches, fatigue, poor memory, mental confusion, learning difficulties, irritability, depression, respiratory ailments, yeast infections, bladder problems, psoriasis, acne, low libido, irregular menses, hormone imbalances, toenail fungus, arthritis, and autism. It can even be involved in such serious illnesses as cancer, AIDS, multiple sclerosis, chronic fatigue syndrome, lupus, and Alzheimer's disease. I would suggest that if you've been diagnosed with one of these labeled diseases, you seek assistance in eradicating chronic candidiasis immediately.

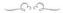

Although there appears to be plenty of evidence to substantiate the existence of candidiasis, traditional mainstream medicine rarely addresses it. Many medical doctors rule out the possibility of candida because its presence isn't always revealed in blood tests or stool cultures, and exists within every human being. But we're aware that fungus is prevalent in epidemic proportions, particularly in North America. Just look at all of the commercials on TV for over-the-counter preparations for toenail fungus, psoriasis, dandruff, anal itching, and vaginal yeast infections. This is not a mystery—it's all about candida albicans and its important link to these seemingly small but irritating problems. I suggest that you locate a skilled medical doctor, naturopathic physician, or holistic practitioner who is familiar with candida and can help you. But keep in mind that unless candida is eradicated *on the inside,* topical skin preparations are only a temporary part of the solution. This reminds me of a classic case I once saw.

Sean's Case

Sean was brought to me when I was teaching a class in medical intuition. I recognized the signs of systemic candidiasis—this rampant yeast condition, which, though internal, had affected the skin all over his body. This 11-month-old baby had eczema, which is almost always associated with candida albicans yeast. Sean had the most severe case I'd ever seen, but fortunately (because I've seen it so often in my clinical days), I wasn't daunted by it. Sean constantly scratched himself to the bleeding point, and he was wearing a white outfit that was so bloodstained that it was almost impossible to look at him. His mother was despondent, and rightfully so. I set about to find out the cause of Sean's frightful eczema.

Sean's mother was of Chinese extraction, and Asian people don't tolerate dairy products due to an enzyme deficiency in their digestive system. Because of his ethnic origin, Sean was allergic to the dairy products he consumed daily. His diet also consisted of plenty of fruit juices, sugars, and fruit—all things candidiasis thrives on.

All fruit, sugars, fruit juices, and dairy products were to be eliminated from Sean's diet for four weeks. The child was under the care of a competent medical doctor and dermatologist, and I suggested that a culture to restore normal bowel bacteria might be helpful. A friend of Sean's mother was a registered nurse who had accompanied them on their visit to me, and she had immediately understood the simple dietary suggestions that I'd made. This woman called me four weeks later to say that Sean was much better. The skin patches were no longer bleeding and were healing nicely.

At that time, I had an instinct that the infant

feeding formula, which was rice based, could still be contributing to the problem. Rice, when it's processed, converts very quickly to sugar in the system, and as I've said, candida yeast thrives on sugar. I suggested that an alternative milk be substituted, and as a two-week experiment, Sean should be given water, combined with appropriate infant vitamin supplementation. Sean is now an active toddler with healthy, clear skin.

Of all the things that I've witnessed in my clinical experience, nothing is more dramatic than the beneficial effects of exterminating this tenacious yeast from the system. An overgrowth of candida albicans isn't difficult to eradicate—remember that candida albicans yeast is fed on starch and sugar in any form. When people eliminate their heavy dependence on these items, this yeast cannot survive, and in approximately one or two months, most of their symptoms dramatically improve. But, as many people are aware, candida does frequently recur and takes a lifetime of careful diligence to see that it's kept under control.

Most people that I see have this yeast as part of their health picture; for instance, an overgrowth of candida can make a person tired, and just about every person I see is exhausted. In a few short weeks of following a candida albicans eradication program, patients are amazed by the return of their energy.

One of the more insidious aspects of this yeast syndrome is that candida albicans can attack healthy brain cells, thus contributing to memory loss. One of the most common complaints and fears that I hear people express is the loss of memory and the experience of "fuzzy thinking." Don't despair, this isn't Alzheimer's disease or old age; it's more likely related to the presence of candida albicans yeast spores, which circulate from the digestive system through the bloodstream. These toxins can affect the delicate balance of the neurological system. After several months of treatment, as the body is detoxified, brain cells can regenerate—I've personally witnessed it.

Imagine that you're taking a walk in a forest and you notice a tall, beautiful tree with a sturdy trunk and branches full of healthy, prolific foliage. Now imagine that you're looking down at the base of the tree and you see what looks like several white dinner plates all joined together, hanging off the side of the trunk. This is a fungus. The tree becomes host to the fungus that lives off of it, and this fungus eventually robs the tree of its vitality. This is the beginning of death for the tree, and so it is in the case of the human being. People with candida are just like trees in the forest. They become the host to the yeasts, fungi, bacteria, or parasites that live inside them. Candida albicans in an overgrowth state is the beginning of death to the human being, and it needs the addiction to sugars of any kind in order to survive. Just like a tree in the forest, a human being doesn't want to be cut down before its time.

On a spiritual level, what is the reason for candidiasis? I believe that most people, on a subconscious level, don't want to be here—they don't want to live. Earth life is hard, and for many people, it's also full of pain. Thus begins the death process. I find it ironic that what pulls us to sugars— that is, their sweet taste—is actually the element that we crave from our work and relationships. When the sweetness of fulfillment in life is missing, we consume it in the form of sugar, which ultimately accelerates the subconscious death wish.

When candida is present, the body's immunity and natural defenses become compromised, and the system eventually breaks down and falls prey to the organisms that live inside it. The solution lies in building up the immune system with positive thoughts and actions, and reducing the sugars and excessive carbohydrates that feed candida yeast.

Next, we'll look at common food allergies and sensitivities and the role that they play in your quest for optimum health.

Common Food Allergies

Along with the identification of candida, probably the single most important factor in a person's health plan is the awareness of their food allergies. As soon as allergic or sensitive foods removed from their diets, most people usually feel a welcome measure of relief.

Certain people develop allergic reactions due to sensitivities to normally harmless substances. This can result in symptoms that affect any part of the body, such as breathing or digestive difficulties, depression, headaches, arthritis, skin rashes, and so on. The range and variety of items to which a person may become sensitive are endless. Sensitivities usually occur after repeated exposure to certain substances. Or, the tendency to become sensitive or allergic to a substance can be inherited. For example, a person may have inherited an intolerance to cows' milk in infancy. But new sensitivities may be added as a result of certain exposures or reactions to a person's environment So, later in life, a lactose-intolerant individual could also acquire an allergy to cat hair after repeated exposure to cats.

There are many common food allergies. Many people are allergic to nuts, particularly peanuts, which can result from a toxic mold. Eggs, tuna, potatoes, corn, citrus fruit, shellfish, and some spices are common allergens. Most people are aware of their immediate allergic reactions—which can result in asthma or skin rashes when exposed to certain airborne inhalants, chemicals, or foods—so these substances are usually avoided in order to prevent severe reactions. But there's also something else worth exploring for people with unsolved chronic problems. Known as *delayed reactions* or *masked food allergies,* these reactions to foods or chemicals aren't always acute or obvious.

It's easy to locate the most common food allergies— take a look at the label of any bottle of vitamins. Right on the label it will probably say, "This product does not contain milk, wheat, corn, yeast or soy." This warning is provided because these items, along with sugar and caffeine, are the most common food allergy culprits. Vitamin companies don't want to take a chance that their supplements will cause allergic reactions.

Food sensitivities almost always occur from the items that you consume on a daily basis. Take a look at what you eat every day. Does your diet include dairy products such as milk, yogurt, cheese, ice cream, or cottage cheese? Dairy is the most common allergen, and many people are sensitive and may have reactions to foods containing it. Common reactions to dairy include gas, bloating, bowel problems, stomach cramps, weight gain, puffy eyes, and sinus and respiratory infections.

Are you consuming products containing wheat? Wheat is the second most common allergen. Wheat or any item made from a sack of flour, in any form, can cause problems related to the joints and bowels, including arthritis, fatigue, puffiness, fluid retention, poor absorption, and heaviness and soreness in the feet or ankles.

(As a side note, it's disheartening to see that almost all of the recipes in every single popular cookbook and almost every woman's magazine contain dairy items or wheat products in some form. There seems to be no escape from these pervasive factors. It's time to wake up and figure it out.)

Corn is another common allergen. Corn, in some form, is found in almost everything that's packaged. Corn sensitivity is usually a factor in people with weight problems.

Sugar, chocolate, and caffeine can trigger nervous system problems and should be avoided. I often see caffeine playing a role in breast lumps or cysts, bladder problems, and in premenstrual tension.

Many people are allergic to soy. For some people, soy is difficult to digest, can block the absorption of iron and other minerals, and there's some evidence to suggest that frequent soy consumption may elevate estrogen levels. High estrogen is often a factor in overweight people, and there's some evidence to indicate that high estrogen levels may contribute to breast cancer. Soy is a legume, a bean. Many people are legume sensitive and have frequent exposure to beans without being aware of it. Coffee, chocolate, and peanuts are all beans in some form.

When I was an allergy tester, the clinic I worked at had a food panel comprised of more than 100 different food items. People were often fascinated by the selection. I always laughed to myself when I tested a person for eel, a fish that relatively few people in North America eat. I figured that one day I would write a song entitled "It's No Big Deal If You're Allergic to Eel"—the principle being that most people are allergic or sensitive to the foods that they eat *every day* and not the strange, uncommon ones.

You may be surprised to know that a person may be allergic to the very substance they're craving. This is why a medical doctor I know suggests to all her patients that for one full week they stop eating all the foods that they usually consume. During this brief period of avoidance, she has found that most of her patients' symptoms subside. Let's take a look at where the desires begin.

Food Allergies and Addictions

Many people are addicted to sugar. I've actually had people break down and cry in front of me when I suggested that for a short period of time, they use an alternative to sugar just to break the cycle. I've found that people crave sugar when they don't consume enough protein. This is particularly true in the case of vegetarians who, unless they're very careful and are aware of protein combinations, tend to consume vast amounts of starch and sugar. (I will further discuss the specific challenges and concerns vegetarians face in Chapter 11.)

When people consume sugar, the pancreas—an organ located just beneath the stomach and responsible for the regulation of blood sugar—releases insulin. When sugar enters the bloodstream, it can trigger the desire in some people for wanting more and more sugar—almost as if the mechanism can't be turned off. A lot of people who desire sugar have widespread candidiasis. When candida is under control, one of the positive benefits is that the sugar cravings subside. Imagine being able to pass a bakery or a candy store without being the slightest bit tempted!

Obese people can identify with the overwhelming power of food addictions. Compulsive eaters continue to consume foods to which they're addicted many times a day. These people, like the drug addict or the alcoholic, have no idea that their daily food cravings are based on a physiological need to prevent the withdrawal symptoms related to their food allergies. The solution for them is to stop consuming the foods that they eat every single day and eat heartily from all the foods they don't eat on a daily basis—until their system has ceased to respond negatively and the immune system is given a chance to recover.

People often ask me how I manage my own cravings. Like many of you, way back in the distant past I was addicted to chocolate chip cookies, bread, and coffee. Chocolate chip cookies would almost seem to call out to me from the freezer to come over, thaw them out, and eat them by the handful. But then, I had the early warning signs of what I thought was a serious illness. It turned out that I had rampant candidiasis and its inherent sweet cravings. I also found out that I was allergic or sensitive to all of the substances that I continually consumed. In environmental medicine, this is what is termed the *addictive/allergic response,* meaning that food-sensitive people can actually crave the foods to which they're allergic. I'll describe this surprising response in detail in the next chapter.

Food Allergies and Immune Reactions

When people have food sensitivities, their body recognizes these substances as foreign invaders. The body reacts to an offending food the same way it reacts to a cold, virus, infection, or bee sting. When someone is stung by a bee, the body's response is to swell up and retain fluid, because the bee's venom is seen as an assailant. Similarly, as soon as a person ingests a food that their body considers an unwelcome attacker, their immune system mobilizes *histamine,* and the person swells up or a part of the body may become inflamed as a result of this *histamine reaction.* Histamine is a substance that's released by the immune system to protect the body and heart from foreign invaders or allergic or toxic substances.

The key is to identify the foods that your body considers foreign invaders, eliminate such foods for a short period of time, let the immune system calm down, and stop initiating histamine reactions. There will almost always be an improvement in symptoms by avoiding the common foods to which you're allergic. After you discover your food sensitivities, how are you going to manage? Guess what? You get to eat other foods more heartily!

Here are some typical questions and answers regarding changing your diet due to food sensitivities.

- *How am I going to manage without wheat and bread? Wheat or flour are everywhere!*

Substitute rice; potatoes; 100 percent rye bread, rye crackers, rice bread, cakes or crackers; sweet potatoes; yams; squash; and unusual grains such as millet, amaranth, quinoa, and buckwheat. Corn can be substituted if it's not an allergen for you.

Avoid wheat to the best of your ability for 30 days. Remember that wheat is wheat is wheat. White bread, brown bread, sprouted wheat—*any* kind of wheat in any form needs to be eliminated. I've also seen wheat-allergic people react to wheat grass and to cosmetics containing wheat germ. While you're avoiding wheat, it can also be helpful to steer clear of oats and barley for the first 30 days, because these are also glutinous grains. After 30 days, these may be reintroduced. Often whole rye, in the form of delicious breads or crackers, can be tolerated because of its low-gluten content. One hundred percent rye bread is delicious toasted or as a base for open-faced sandwiches. There are many wheat-free breads, pastas, and cookies available in most health-food stores.

After your 30-day avoidance program, you may introduce wheat on an occasional basis, such as once every fifth day. This process is called *rotation*, a procedure that avoids the overexposure of a food or substance and prevents the body from becoming allergic or sensitive to that substance.

- *How am I going to manage without dairy products?*

Dairy products are much easier to avoid than wheat products. Dairy products are always a choice—that is, you're either pouring the milk, cutting the cheese, or spooning out the ice cream.

Try using soy milk, rice milk, or almond milk in your cereal. You system may tolerate goats' milk and cheese and sheep's cheese. For children or adults who have sinus problems, goats' milk or any other alternative milks may aggravate their symptoms. Some people may experience problems from drinking cows' *milk,* but cheese, yogurt or cultured cows' milk *products* may be tolerated.

- *Will I ever be able to eat wheat or dairy products again?*

Of course, as long as you remember not to ingest the offending items frequently—no more than every fifth day—on a rotation basis.

- *Because of candida, I'm avoiding sugars and juice. What do I do for sweets?*

Good question. Usually a person who craves starches and sugars needs more protein. You should try choosing protein for a snack, as it will "hold" you longer. For a sweet treat, try a rice cake with a tiny scraping of honey on it. Alternative sweeteners such as Stevia (a natural herbal sweetener) and Splenda® or Sucralose® (an altered sugar, used in diet foods and low-carbohydrate snacks) are available in grocery and health-food stores.

NutraSweet®, or aspartame, is a synthesized sweetener made from an amino acid combination. It's widely used in diet foods and soft drinks, and has received much negative press lately. However, speaking as an allergy tester, this sugar substitute rarely showed up as a problem except in hyperactive children or for people with chemical sensitivities. Personally, I notice that my throat feels dry when I chew gum containing this substance. Trust your own guidance when using anything but a natural sweetener. I feel that sugar substitutes can be an important temporary transition away from excess cravings and sugar consumption. But just knowing that your cravings for sweets will diminish after your candida is eradicated is one of the positive benefits.

- *What about my children?*

If your child is dairy sensitive, look for an appropriate milk substitute. Remember that after a period of avoidance in order to clear symptoms, your child should be able to enjoy dairy products occasionally on a rotation basis.

In the meantime, try rice ice cream, tofu ice cream, or all-fruit sorbet—they're sweet, delicious alternatives to "traditional" ice cream. Feed your children adequately at each meal, and cut down on sugar and "junk" items. Nuts also make good snacks.

- *What about alcohol?*

Remember that this plan is for a short period of time, while your body rebalances—it usually only takes 30 days. But ideally, if you're eradicating candida albicans, then wine and beer need to be avoided because they're fermented beverages that also contain yeasts. But hard liquor is usually allowed because it's distilled, so the occasional ounce may be permissible. If you're working on a candida yeast eradication program, any sort of fermented food should be avoided, including cheese, mushrooms, soy sauce, pickles, and vinegar. (More information regarding ferments is found in the Environmental Illness section on page 95.) Headaches or postnasal drip are common symptoms associated with yeast or mold sensitivity.

- *What happens after 30 days?*

Usually you'll experience a noticeable improvement in your health. Most of the complaints you had 30 days ago will be greatly diminished. You'll be able to eat the offending foods on a rotation basis—I call this plan "three sins a week." In other words, you can enjoy a sweet dessert, a glass of wine, an exposure to dairy products, or another "no-no" food three times per week, and your body will probably say, "Fine, I can handle that!" However, overexposure to offending foods may cause your symptoms to return.

- *Will I ever be clear of these allergies?*

Yes, when you relieve your body of stress and work consistently on your emotional issues. In the meantime, a period of avoidance is the most practical solution in order to relieve pressure from the immune system. You might consider investigating homeopathy, a cleansing program, allergy desensitizing techniques, or neutralizing drops (found through an environmental medical clinic) for relief.

(For more in-depth information regarding the day-to-day management of food allergies, refer to *A Basic Food Plan* on page 259. This simple plan, which usually works well for most people, will round out your knowledge and answer more of your questions. It will also give you tips for snacks, traveling, and dining out.)

There are some people who are very rigid about the kinds of food they'll eat. Some people are interested in food combining, some only eat raw foods, some people "fast" or stop eating solid foods for a few days on occasion, and some eat only fruits or vegetables. There are many plans and many ways for people to eat—no *one* way works for everyone. You'll find out what's best for you when you learn to tune in to your body and find out what *it* really wants.

As I tell people, if you're feeling like a million bucks on the program that you're currently following, then it's the right program for you. If you're not feeling energetic and fabulously healthy, then it may be time to reevaluate your program.

In the next chapter, we'll cover all of the components of a successful weight-loss program. Even if you don't need to lose weight, by reading this chapter, you'll glean many hints that can increase your overall level of health.

Chapter 6

Weight Issues

When I see overweight men and women poring over diet meals in the freezer case at the grocery store, I find this very sad. These "diet" entrees feature small portions in fancy packages; and they advertise that they contain minimal calories, no fat, and no cholesterol—but they're loaded guns. These meals don't help overweight people in their quest to lose weight. In fact, such meals can often hinder them in their quest for better health due to the incredibly high levels of salt and chemicals—*and* they contain allergic foods!

Most people don't realize how simple it is to lose weight. Contrary to popular belief, losing weight isn't about counting calories, weighing food on scales, measuring portions, or starvation. It's about knowing what the body wants, and how it utilizes certain foods and translates them into cell tissue—particularly those foods that it's allergic to. I call this the great fat/fluid myth.

Let's look at the common components of the weight issue.

1. **Food allergies**—Almost all overweight people have food allergies, particularly to common foods that are eaten every day. This includes candidiasis, which can trigger tremendous cravings for starches and sugars. Most overweight people are afflicted with candida, but it's easy to correct.

2. **Excessive carbohydrate consumption**—Carbohydrates (starches) convert quickly to sugar. Excess sugar is converted to fat and stored in the cells, leading to weight gain.

3. **Hormone imbalances**—Another major component of the weight issue is hormones. Overweight people often have thyroid and related endocrine problems. Hormones require careful balancing.

4. **Exercise**—Overweight people need to get their bodies and lymphatic systems moving, tune and tone up their muscles and fibers, increase their heart rates, and simply feel better. They should pick a simple activity that they can commit to every day.

5. **Bowel movements**—Believe it or not, this is a very telling area regarding weight loss. If the body is holding on to excess matter (resulting in constipation), this can contribute to weight gain. Conversely, a case of diarrhea means that the body isn't getting a chance to absorb nutrients.

Following are some useful guidelines if you're ten pounds or more overweight.

Food Allergies and Weight Gain

Most people aren't aware that the foods they consume on a daily basis can actually be their biggest enemy. This is true for both weight loss and the quest for better health. Many suffer from what is termed an *addictive/allergic response.* This means that people can actually be allergic to the foods they crave, and must eat these foods in order to stave off withdrawal symptoms. Food allergies (or sensitivities) engage the immune system, which recognizes certain foods (particularly dairy, and wheat or flour products) as foreign invaders. The body reacts defensively against the allergen and engages the immune system. A chemical called histamine is released, and it can induce tissue damage, inflammation, and fluid retention. This fluid is stored in the body's tissue, rather like a filing cabinet. The body says, "I don't like what she/he's consuming, so I'm going to store this in the tissue until I can figure it out later."

Unfortunately, this never happens. The body never can "figure it out later" because the person keeps consuming the same foods, which can be aggravating the system day after day. As soon as the person stops consuming the offending foods, the body miraculously releases the stored fluid, and it's urinated out of the body.

Food-sensitive people tend to crave foods that release serotonin, the "feel-good" chemical in the brain. They usually gravitate toward sugars and refined carbohydrates, which give them a similar "high." But this temporary feeling of well-being invariably leads to a decline in blood-sugar levels, resulting in fatigue and a myriad of other undesirable symptoms. As soon as the North American diet industry understands this simple concept and everyone becomes aware of their own individual food allergies and sensitivities, the entire business will be revolutionized.

―◌◌―

One big myth most overweight people mistakenly believe is that there are certain foods that will help them lose weight because they're low in calories. One such food that falls into this category is cottage cheese—this, or any low-fat cheese, is a staple in the diet industry. How many people start a diet on Monday morning with a plate of low-fat cottage cheese and fruit? But cottage cheese is a dairy product, and dairy, although delicious, can trigger immune reactions. So the body recognizes the cottage cheese, low-fat or otherwise, as an attacker, mobilizes histamine, and stores the resulting fluid in the body. As soon as people identify their food allergies and stop creating histamine reactions, they won't be storing fluid in the tissue—thus, they'll lose weight.

If you want to slim down, I suggest that you stop consuming dairy or wheat products, sugar in any form, and caffeine for a period of four weeks. If you're suspicious about corn—which can be a common allergen in overweight people—avoid *it* as well. Corn in some form is almost always contained in baked goods or processed foods, and because it's so sweet and breaks down to sugar so quickly, it can contribute to carbohydrate and blood-sugar problems.

Next, take a look at your legume (bean) consumption. Legumes, although tasty, can be hard to digest, contributing to gas and bloating. Peanuts and soybeans are legumes; coffee and chocolate belong to different *food families* (see page 277), but they're also a variety of bean. And don't forget about soy—it's the fifth most common food allergy and is a much-used filler in the production of many packaged foods. Soy can contribute to an increase in estrogen production, and overweight people often have high estrogen levels. The current popularity of soy consumption may not be appropriate for every body. Leave soy and beans in any form out of your diet for four weeks. Use your instincts to detect which of these foods could be involved in your weight problems.

So what are you going to eat? You're going to *eat heartily from everything else.* Imagine being able to lose weight without measuring out portions, starving, and counting calories. What a relief!

The Carbohydrate Equation

Now let's talk about carbohydrates, another important element of weight loss. After you've identified all your food sensitivities and have eliminated them for approximately 30 days, the next step is to analyze your carbohydrate or starch intake. There are several popular books on the market that discuss the low-carbohydrate diet. These books can be very useful in explaining how cholesterol is formed, and how a low-carbohydrate diet can lower blood pressure, and they can help diabetic and pre-diabetic conditions. An excellent reference for following a low-carbohydrate plan is *Protein Power* (Bantam, 1997) by a medical doctor husband-and-wife team, Mary Dan and Michael Eades.

The basic principle of the low-carbohydrate program is that you don't eat starches such as breads, pasta, cakes, cookies, popcorn, rice, or potatoes in excess. The plan focuses on the consumption of animal protein; or protein from beans, legumes, nuts, and seeds, as well as plenty of vegetables and some fruit in moderation. (First, make sure you use your intuition to parse out food sensitivities.) Portions of the above foods aren't limited; it's just the carbohydrates (starches) that are measured—now you *do* have to start counting. A low-carbohydrate program suggests that you consume approximately 30 grams of carbohydrates for the first two weeks and 60 grams after that. I find that 60 grams of carbohydrates per day from the onset of a low-carbohydrate program is a manageable amount. (See "An Easy-to-Follow Carbohydrate Plan" on page 69.)

Here's the basic principle of a low-carbohydrate plan. Let's say that for breakfast, you eat two whole-grain muffins loaded with fiber, honey, dried fruit, and molasses—very healthy, right? Well, as soon as you start eating those muffins, they begin to convert to sugar in your digestive system. In less than an hour, there's approximately one cup of sugar speeding around in your bloodstream. Then the pancreas, the organ that regulates blood sugar, goes to work and releases insulin to take care of this rise in blood sugar—all of this the result of the two "healthy" muffins.

At the same time that the pancreas is taking care of the rise in blood sugar, it also gives a message to the liver to create cholesterol in the same amount. Cholesterol is stored in the body unless it's used up through exertion (exercise). The trick with a low-carbohydrate diet is to not initiate a strong insulin response from the pancreas. This way, the pancreas isn't overworked, constantly releasing insulin, nor is it constantly giving messages to the liver to create cholesterol.

Also keep in mind that it can be useful to avoid caffeine when following a low-carbohydrate plan. Caffeine stimulates a temporary surge in blood sugar, which can be followed by an overproduction of insulin and a low-blood-sugar downward spiral.

A low-carbohydrate plan can be very effective. Not only do people have more energy (because they're not consuming sugars and excessive starches), but they tend to lower their cholesterol and blood pressure, and sometimes are able to even reduce or discontinue diabetes medication. When there's very little sugar in the blood, cravings appear to subside, and the body uses up the stored fat in the tissues for fuel. Weight loss naturally follows.

Pity all those poor people who've been avoiding fats and animal proteins—neither of which trigger an insulin response—and have been consuming excessive amounts of carbohydrate, which *does* trigger an insulin response, in an effort to lose weight.

—◌◌—

With all due respect to the low-carbohydrate diet books out there, they're all missing one important element—food allergies and sensitivities. Almost all of these books encourage people to eat cream, cheese, sour cream, and cottage cheese in liberal amounts. Remember, the number-one food sensitivity for most people with weight and assorted health problems is dairy products. It baffles me that no one has figured out this obvious connection. When people have been on a low-carbohydrate diet and have reached a plateau or haven't lost a significant amount of weight, I encourage them to avoid dairy products for several weeks. I especially urge DLH types (with their tendency toward lymphatic blockages) to follow this advice. Usually the reduction of dairy will be the linchpin, and the weight starts to drop off.

Plan to keep your carbohydrate intake to approximately 60 grams per day. It can also be helpful to avoid eating fruit or carbohydrates at breakfast and lunch so that insulin levels aren't increased during those times, and there's no subsequent crash in blood-sugar levels. Save the carbohydrates for dinner, when a drop in blood sugar and energy won't affect late-day activities. Many people find that if they eat carbohydrates—even fruit or a small amount of starch—at breakfast or lunch, they continue to crave these sweets and starches for the rest of the day. Experiment with this yourself. Your body is the laboratory, and it will show you the effects of what you're doing.

An Easy-to-Follow Carbohydrate Plan

Here's an easy guideline to follow. I consider it a little rigid, but it can be a useful kick-start to following a low-carbohydrate plan. Your aim for the first two weeks is to keep your carbohydrate intake at approximately 30 grams per day. At the end of two weeks, I suggest that you increase your daily carbohydrate gram intake to 60 grams per day and expand your food horizons at this time.

You can eat any amount of meat, fish, poultry, and eggs (providing you have no sensitivities to these items). Butter, nuts, and oils may also be used sparingly. If you do *not* have allergies or sensitivities to dairy products, then cheese, milk, and cream may be consumed in limited amounts as well.

I don't calculate the carbohydrate in vegetables as part of the 60-gram total, except for carrots, beets, and other sweet, starchy vegetables. Keep your intake of starchy vegetables low. For example: 1 cup cooked winter squash = 10 grams of carbohydrate, and 1 medium-sized sweet potato = 20 grams of carbohydrates. (See the list on page 288.) Choose green vegetables, as they're low in carbohydrates, and you can eat an unlimited amount.

Vegetable Choices

- Eat any amount of the following vegetables, cooked or raw: arugula, asparagus, bean sprouts, bok choy, broccoli, cabbage, cauliflower, celery, collard greens, crookneck squash, cucumber, endive, escarole, fresh herbs, green pepper, kale, kohlrabi, lettuce, pattypan squash, parsley, radishes, spinach, su choy, summer squash, watercress, zucchini.

Starchy Vegetable Choices

- For the first two weeks of your program, keep your consumption of these vegetables low (refer to the carbohydrate list for verification): artichokes, avocado, beets, Brussels sprouts, butternut squash, carrots, Danish squash, eggplant, jicama, leeks, okra, olives, onion, pumpkin, sweet potatoes, tomatoes, turnips, water chestnuts, winter squash, yams.

Beverages

- Limit your beverage intake to these items (which you can have an unlimited supply of): herbal or decaffeinated teas or coffee, coffee substitutes, beef or chicken broth, and purified water.

Fruit

- Consume fresh fruit on a limited basis—as snacks only—and watch the carbohydrate grams.

Here's a surprising look at some carbohydrate grams.

- 1 slice bread = 20–25 grams
- 1 medium potato = 20 grams
- 1 cup cooked rice = 20 grams
- 1 ear of corn = 20 grams
- 2 RyKrisp® (whole rye) crackers = 14 grams
- 1 rice cake = 8–13 grams
- 15 almonds or ¼ cup = 5 grams
- ½ avocado = 5 grams

Refer to the carbohydrate gram chart on page 288 or to low-carbohydrate diet books for a complete list of foods and information.

Hormones

When I look into a physical body, I see it in terms of the systems that are out of balance, and one of the most common areas of imbalance occurs in the endocrine system. All too often, people can blame themselves, their emotional issues, or their past experiences, when much of their mental anguish can actually stem from endocrine imbalances. Overweight people almost always have hormone imbalances; and in my own life as a menopausal woman, I know that my emotional well-being has been greatly enhanced by using a natural hormone formula.

I remember seeing an elderly woman, long past her menopausal years, who could not stop crying. She cried off and on from morning till night. This had been her problem for five years, and her husband was at a loss as to what to do for her. She'd been to doctors, psychiatrists, and many practitioners trying to find a solution to her constant weeping.

This woman had an endocrine problem—fortunately, I knew of a medical doctor who specialized in hormone imbalances using subtle methods of treatment. I felt this would be useful. By pinpointing the exact area of imbalance and providing the specific remedy to treat it, she was able to find relief at last.

Men will often come to me with low testosterone levels. I wonder why, on an energetic level, this sex hormone can be so low. Could this hormone be subconsciously suppressed in some men due to women becoming more powerful and confident in the world? Again, appropriate hormone balance will assist men and women (we all produce testosterone) in regaining energy, well-being, and libido.

The candida yeast syndrome, which I've discussed at length in these pages, can often contribute to a low-functioning thyroid. The thyroid gland, located at the base of the neck, is involved in maintaining body-weight balance, body temperature, energy, and overall well-being. It's very often out of balance; in fact, some doctors say that there is thyroid imbalance in epidemic proportions in this country. People with low-functioning thyroids will often have difficulty losing weight, and a medical test may not always detect it. On an energetic level, I see a person with a low-functioning thyroid gland as heavy, sluggish, dark, and gray. They'll often look oily, unwashed, and unclean to me—even if they just took a shower.

The use of certain herbs, botanicals, glandular materials, or synthetic thyroid medication will help this important gland to function correctly. For many people, it's as if the lights finally go on and the afterburners for energy and weight loss go up after the thyroid is balanced. For instance, take a look at this letter I recently received from Fred, a 50-year-old man who had a lifelong battle with his weight.

> *"Since I saw you in the summer of 2000, I've lost 48 pounds. I followed your food-allergy avoidance program, eradicating candida yeast and improving my thyroid function. You helped me to demystify my body's processes. I no longer wake up with a stuffy nose and headaches, my body doesn't hurt, and I have five times more energy than I did before. I'm very grateful to you, Caroline."*

If a people are trying to lose weight and they're following all of the appropriate guidelines relating to food allergies, limiting carbohydrate grams, and exercising daily, yet they've reached a plateau in their quest for the ideal body weight, it usually points to a hormone imbalance. It takes a person with a great deal more knowledge than I have in this regard to assist them. However, there are naturally based supplements, as well as prescription medications available, which can help. When it comes to hormones, seek help from a competent practitioner.

The Benefits of Exercise

Along with any health or weight-loss program, exercise is a key component. "Ugh," you say. Don't despair, the dreaded "E word" isn't that bad. When the word *exercise* is mentioned, most people conjure up an image of hours of sweating at the gym, or they're terrified to even go to the gym for fear of exposing their out-of-shape bodies to others.

When I'm with a client, I get a sense of what kind of exercise would benefit them the most. In a CNS type, steady, rhythmic exercise such as tai chi, yoga, or swimming might be more beneficial than what they're currently doing, which may be nothing at all or something too strenuous. CNS people can be calmed through the action of slow, focused exercise, incorporating specific movements that require being in the present moment. DLH types would probably respond to boxing, Tae-Bo, weightlifting, or running, since these are activities that get them "unstuck" and moving.

Most of the time, when I tune in to people, more intense exercise on a cardiovascular level seems to be required. In the case of overweight or out-of-shape people, I usually hear a loud groan when cardiovascular exercise is mentioned, and the thought of a sweaty body pounding it out on the pavement brings terror to their hearts. None of this is necessary.

Let's tune in to the body and see what it really wants. If you close your eyes for a second and ask yourself what type of exercise would be beneficial for your body, you might be quite surprised.

I led a friend through this exercise at her lakeside home. She'd always been a distance runner, but now that she was in her early 60s, she felt that running was too hard on her body. Going to the gym, however, wasn't appealing to her at all. In meditation, she received the impression that rowing would be good for her. In all the years she'd lived by the lake, she'd never thought of engaging in this activity. She purchased a beautiful wooden rowboat, and every day she takes in the scenery around the lake, along with enjoying a wonderful cardiovascular workout.

When you tune in to the body in this manner, let the wisdom come from within. Because the instincts of your body are directly linked to what will give you the most joy and the best exercise—like my friend with the rowboat—an unexpected form of exercise might be revealed. It could be tap dancing, swimming, Pilates, or ballet, as well as any "traditional" form of exercise.

I remember doing a late-night radio interview in Los Angeles. I got a strong sense that the caller I was speaking to was out of balance, largely from lack of exercise. This man was a night owl, which made sense, as he was calling the program well past midnight. From the sound of his voice, I had a sense that swimming would be a peaceful, worthwhile experience for him and would balance the hours that he spent at his computer. He later reported that he looked forward to his daily swim, noticing how out of touch with nature he'd become over the years.

I suggest to people that they lace up their athletic shoes and walk every day for about 15 minutes. If you're a CNS type, this will help you alleviate pent-up frustrations. If you're a DLH person, the action of walking will help stimulate the lymphatic system in the removal of toxins from your body.

Every so often during your walk, put on a "head of steam"—power-walk or walk like a duck for about 20 to 30 paces. Pick a marker—perhaps a tree or a telephone pole—

and power-walk to that marker. Swing your arms, quicken your pace, and increase your heart rate. Just travel as far as you're comfortable. Every few days, add another segment of power walking to your daily walk. In a few weeks, you might even feel like a comfortable jog during one of these jaunts. The idea is to get the heart rate up, improve the function of the lymphatic system, and increase those "feel-good" brain chemicals into the body, which curb hunger pangs and improve attitude.

I remember when I met Marnie. She weighed approximately 300 pounds. It was difficult to help her because she was one of The Tricky People. Even so, every day she put on her shoes and walked, which was an arduous task for her. At first, she could only walk around the block; then it increased to two blocks. Within six weeks, she had lost 20 pounds and could walk a mile. The first thing she did after she got up in the morning was to take that walk. Exercise is a huge component in weight loss, as well as physical and mental well-being.

If you have exercise equipment, use your treadmill or exercise bike for five minutes a day for one or two weeks, then increase to five minutes twice daily. The body knows what you're doing and will respond. Resist the temptation in the beginning to think that you have to exercise long and hard. Just do something.

I often recommend the use of a rebounder or mini-trampoline, which can be a fun cardiovascular exercise, and is also less taxing to muscles and joints. It seems that in this weightless state, as the body jumps, there may be benefits to the lymphatic system. Use the rebounder for three minutes per day for the first ten days, and then increase to three minutes twice a day and build up.

Bowel Movements

On the physical level, there's almost no other quest that's as important as the search for the perfect bowel movement. Often people with weight problems suffer from constipation. Imagine packing all that extra waste material around! On an emotional level, constipation often relates to letting go of anger and past issues. It can be a factor in people with control or perfectionist tendencies as well.

After all of my all years as an allergy-testing technician, picking up the test vials for gut linings, large intestines, rectums, and anuses day after day, I can safely say that almost every person I tested was unbalanced in one or more of these areas. In the world of environmental medicine, the intestinal tract is the command post of the human body. What goes on *in* and *into* the gut can affect the entire machine. Bowel movements are interesting and necessary. I spend a lot of time intuitively (thank God) "scoping out" people's bowel movements.

"Constipation of the Nation" could be the name of another song that I should write. It's such a common problem. People can go for *days* without going to the bathroom. In fact, I remember one woman telling me that she only had a bowel movement once a month!

I also suffered from chronic constipation for many years until I was tested for food allergies. Wheat, or anything that was made from a sack of flour (that included all my favorite foods), made me constipated. Dairy products also had the same effect on me. As soon as I removed these foods from my diet, except for the occasional exposure, I was no longer constipated. Candida yeast, because it lines the intestinal tract, is well known for its contribution to constipation.

Physically, constipation involves several factors. We have to take food allergies into consideration, balance intestinal flora, make sure water intake is adequate, and supply plenty of fiber and roughage to the diet. Liver and gall bladder functions need to be supported, and hormones also need to be looked at—often a low-functioning thyroid and a sluggish liver can cause constipation. Everyone is different—one equation might work for one person and not for another.

_____

On the other side of the coin are the people who have loose bowel movements or diarrhea. The foods they eat never stay in their intestinal tract long enough for the nutrients to be absorbed. These people are often pale and tired and can be very thin, anemic, and lacking in stamina.

For the most part, this isn't a mystery—take a look at what you eat. Everything you ingest has an effect on your intestinal tract and bowel movements. Take a seven-day experiment and leave everything aside that you currently eat and drink, and eat heartily from everything else, noticing your bowel movements along the way.

People who have loose bowel movements, just like those who are constipated, need to take a good look at wheat—a common culprit—and dairy products, which can often trigger a flow of loose fecal material. Sugar also needs to be paid attention to—in fact, it's probably the worst offender. The goal is to slow the bowel movement down so that it passes through the intestinal tract more slowly, allowing the nutrients to be absorbed. The following are two examples of people with bowel movement problems.

Corey's Case

Corey, a man in his 30s, was a college student; consequently, he had almost no money and no medical doctor. He had loose bowel movements, sometimes like water, and a bleeding rectum. It would be a daunting prospect to help a man in this condition, so I urged him to see a medical doctor, to no avail. I agreed to work with him for two weeks if he would promise to go to a doctor.

When a person has loose bowel movements, the lower colon can be very irritated. Any husky grain, such as whole wheat, corn, or even brown rice, can aggravate the problem. Because Corey was a student, he lived on brown rice. I suggested that for three days he eat the following at every meal: acorn squash, steamed green vegetables, and chicken or fish, which he'd cook himself. If his colon ceased to be irritated, I told him, the bleeding would stop.

At the time, I was doing consultations in a large Victorian house near the campus Corey attended. I was swamped with clients, so I instructed him to leave a note under my door describing his progress. After three days, he did drop me a line verifying my instincts—his bleeding had indeed stopped. I called him and said he should continue the regime without change for another three days. Once again, I got the same report from him—no bleeding.

We then adjusted the program and added some low-gluten rice and medicinal tea to the equation, which can strengthen the lower colon. To this day, as long as Corey stays away from husky grains, particularly wheat and corn, his bowel movements are normal. (And he did see a medical doctor as promised.)

Dan's Case

Dan sought my help for a problem very similar to Corey's. It was scary for me to think that there was blood in the toilet every time he had a bowel movement. He was a struggling house painter whose diet consisted mainly of doughnuts and colas, and he also had no medical doctor. I agreed to work with him for two weeks if he promised to seek medical attention and have the appropriate colon tests. I suggested the same regime for Dan as I did for Corey—with one difference.

By looking at the pale color of his face and the limp, dry quality of his hair, I knew that Dan's nutritional absorption had to be poor. Looking at his small intestine confirmed my suspicions. So my instincts told me that he should take his mealtime nourishment as a soup. Soups are readily tolerated by the body, especially if the ingredients don't include items to which the person is sensitive. I suggested a basic chicken soup, substituting squash, which is very easily tolerated, for noodles. Green vegetables, chicken stock, and chunks of chicken were added to the mix. This hearty brew, I suggested, should be consumed at every meal for three days.

At the end of the three-day experiment, Dan called me to say that his bowel movements had slowed down from being jet propelled, and that there was no more blood in the toilet. We were on the right track.

I suggested that he continue the soup plan for another three days, alternating between chicken and fish for variety. He reported back that not only were the bowel movements settling down, but his stamina was improving as well. His body was absorbing the nutrition in the soup and reflecting this positive benefits back to him. This carried on for another three-day cycle—he was getting bored with the regime but it was working.

Then we expanded Dan's food horizons and added in one item at a time, noting any changes in his bowel movements. At last report, he's almost back to normal with his diet, except he continues to avoid wheat products, doughnuts, and colas.

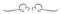

From these stories, you can see the dramatic role that certain foods play, both in the realm of weight loss and in our overall health picture. Many overweight people are bored with life and are waiting for something to happen. Often, they have a strong little child inside them, which constantly requires food to feel better. Let's move on to the deep and poignant topic of addictions and how they affect us on many levels.

Chapter 7

Understanding Addictions

Many ill people have obvious patterns of addiction or low self-esteem running through their lives. An addiction is anything that has a "hold" on us, such as work, exercise, sex, food (especially chocolate, sugar, and coffee), alcohol, cigarettes, illegal drugs, medications, money, worry, material possessions, relationships, negativity, overachieving, gambling, and so on. People can even be addicted to illness.

These addictive tendencies begin in childhood with our constant need for attention. Our parents or caregivers kept us quiet with food, the breast or bottle, pacifiers, toys, outings, and other diversions. The minute we squawked, we were given something to keep us quiet. Now that we're adults, we rely upon our addictions to numb the pain and frustration of daily existence. Our addictions give us a sense of power and control over our random, workaday lives.

Coffee drinkers, for example, can describe in minute detail the feeling of their special brand of elixir as it touches every inch of their alimentary tract. And yet, you wouldn't believe the number of people seeking optimum health while being addicted to caffeine, chocolate, and sugars—not to mention illegal drugs, cigarettes, and alcohol. Obviously, as soon as people stop taking these addictive substances, their health dramatically improves.

Seeing Addictions from a Spiritual Point of View

Some people have had very traumatic childhoods, and the comfort that their bad habits provide is justifiable. But the grapple hook of addictions can be an avoidance mechanism to take people off the path toward fulfillment, or can prevent them from exploring issues and subjects that expose their vulnerability. I believe that life is all about learning, growing, and mastering certain behaviors, the least of which are addictions.

On a higher, spiritual level, addictions are interesting. They have great power over us, and also carry negative vibrations, which can be seen energetically. These negative energies or "entities" attach themselves to the physical body. When I see an addicted person, I can tell that something has a hold on them. I will see black all around the person—they appear unclear or dark, as if they're engulfed in a murky cloud. Some negative force is sapping their life force or vitality—and I know that they're addicted.

From the spiritual perspective, *nothing* can have a hold on us—no substance, person, place, or possession. We must be free, clear, and available to be moved by the universe. Addictions derail us and keep us from fully entering life and heeding our true callings. Staying stuck in a bad habit of any kind means that we're not really ready to grow up and take full responsibility for the life that God has given us.

Another way of putting it is if we're addicted, we're not clear. We don't give off lucent, radiant energy from our bodies; therefore, our auras (or electromagnetic fields) are muddy. The emission of brilliant, pure energy from our physical selves is significant in the area of *manifestation;*

that is, we desire to attract the best to us on a material and spiritual level. I believe that exuding this luminous energy is the cornerstone to materializing positive experiences. A clear and healthy physical body, and plenty of personal fulfillment, is necessary for optimum health. If we're blocked in *any* way, whether it's due to addiction or illness, our physical bodies become tired and worn down, and we cannot reach our highest potential.

Emotions and Cravings

On an emotional level, an addicted person has a very strong little child inside of them who's running the show. "Life is too difficult, and I must have my treats, my pacifier, or something to make me feel better," this child says. When people realize that the body they've been given is an instrument to carry them through to complete their mission and purpose in this life, they then seem happy to let go of their unhealthy cravings and addictions in favor of a healthier lifestyle.

I'm often asked how I manage my own food cravings. Like many of you, I have a formidable inner child that needs plenty of nurturing. I have to let the little child have her treats—treats that won't make me feel sick. Because I'm very aware of my food sensitivities, I had to do a lot of research and recipe-tweaking in order to find goodies that wouldn't make my candidiasis proliferate, spike my blood sugar (which would give me that tired, low-energy feeling later on), or initiate a histamine reaction, which would trigger food allergies.

On occasion, I do enjoy a sweet dessert or a glass of wine. I indulge myself occasionally, but it has to be something really special. For instance, for a delectable slice of hazelnut torte or a dish of crème brûlée, I might be willing to pay the price of feeling a little "off" the next day. But it's not worth it for me to jeopardize my whole program just for a mundane piece of pie or an ordinary cookie. When, like me, you know your body so well that you can tell when it's slightly left of center, the foods that you used to crave will no longer have a hold on you. The value that you'll place on a finely tuned, healthy body will just be too great.

Addiction to Medication

I can't stress enough the importance of competent, regular medical attention. The use of medication is between you and your doctor. There's a place for medication, just as there's a place for natural remedies—everything works together. Thanks to medication, hearts are regulated, diabetes is controlled, headaches are cured, and pain is alleviated.

But there are people who are overmedicated and will reach for "magic bullets" whenever a symptom of any kind appears. That is, they're addicted to the concept of taking medication for every ailment that they have, instead of trying to figure out where the problem originated. On some level, people can often be addicted to the emotional drama that they've created in their lives, and they prefer to look to medication as a remedy, instead of dealing with what caused the pain in the first place. When a person is medicated, this presents an interesting challenge for me intuitively. When I tune in to a body, it normally looks like a road map to me—but when someone is medicated or especially overmedicated, I can't see the "map" because it's covered with clouds. Much like a person with any kind of addiction, the medicated person appears not to be a "real" person, but someone wearing a disguise, which masks who they are on a physical level.

Inge's Case

Forty-year-old Inge came to me seeking help. She was on eight different medications, and I could hardly look at her body intuitively. Energetically, she was as scattered and discordant as an orchestra with every single member playing off-key. Her body was laboring under the strain of trying to deal with all of these medications. She took antidepressants and hormone-balancing medication, as well as pills for sleep, to prevent asthma attacks, and for high blood pressure. On the surface, she appeared to be a bright, positive person, but underneath, she was dealing with plenty of emotional issues.

Every day, she drank coffee and ate copious amounts of dairy products, to which she was obviously allergic. She was also addicted to chocolate. Yet, even at 50 pounds overweight, Inge seemed very motivated and anxious to conquer her health issues, and although I was skeptical and reluctant, I agreed to work with her.

We identified her food allergies and checked out her home for environmental factors that might have been triggering her asthma. I suggested simple supplementation to support her body, and emotional counseling for her soul. (The reduction of her medications was between her and her doctor.) Today, Inge has lost weight, no longer has asthma attacks, and has greatly reduced her medication.

Paulette's Case

People are often addicted to their illnesses. The experience of being in pain can bring great rewards in terms of care, nurturing, and most important—love.

Paulette is a perfect example of someone who used illness in an addictive manner to gain the attention and helpful concern of her husband. When I met Paulette, her chronic illness was the center of her focus. But as is the case with many people I work with, I knew that Paulette didn't *have* to be ill. She walked with a cane and was obviously in a great deal of pain, yet I knew intuitively that her body had every capacity to be fully functional.

I suggested a very simple program of food allergy avoidance, yeast eradication, and supplementation. Two days later, I had the opportunity to see her again at a medical intuitive training session. In the 48 hours since I'd first seen her, she was able to get out of a chair without help. I was fascinated—how could this body that was so out of balance start to correct itself so quickly? I decided to keep track of Paulette's progress, and I called her a week later. She continued to improve and had gained more mobility. She joked that she might even have to go back to work.

A month later, I placed a follow-up call. She'd slipped back into her old habits and addictions. Why wouldn't Paulette want to help herself and recover? The price of losing her doting husband's constant care and attention, coupled with the looming possibility of returning to work, was just too much for her to contend with.

It's sad that so many people forget this basic concept: The body knows what to do to get healthy. Paulette's brief glimpse at a level of wellness that she'd only dreamed about confirms this important truth. Optimum health takes a deeper level of commitment than some people are willing to make, and as a medical intuitive, I find that the unraveling of this multilayered puzzle can be both disturbing and rewarding. It's very sad for me to watch the grip that addictions have on some people, and how they can never reach their best health—physically or emotionally—until they come to terms with their "demons."

In the next chapter, we'll discuss the impact of emotional and physical issues on our body's framework or structure.

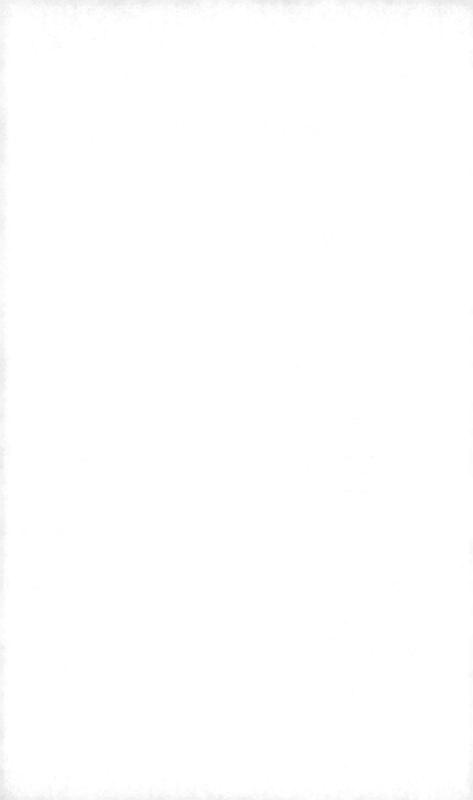

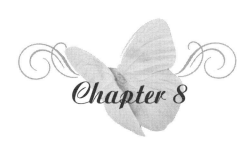

Chapter 8

Bones and Skeletons

I'm going to include a very brief chapter on skeletal imbalances, since I don't usually "see" them. My instincts aren't trained in this manner, and it doesn't appear to be my domain. My aptitude lies in perceiving the organs and organ systems in the body, as well as the environmental factors we've been addressing. So, I prefer to leave the skeletal structure to the practitioners who have expertise in that area. However, when organs, systems, and processes are supplied with proper nutrition, the skeletal system is also nourished. Toxins circulating around in the bloodstream can hinder the supply of nourishment to the bones.

People are often delightfully surprised when, simply by reducing body toxins, their stiff necks ease, the pain in their lower back improves, and their muscles become more flexible. Many people comment about the suppleness of their necks and joints after several weeks on a specific toxic-reducing program. One woman remarked that for the first time in years, she was able to turn her head comfortably to the side during her square-dancing classes.

Countless people complain of lower back pain. Often their bulging waistlines are putting great pressure on their back muscles. In most cases, once these people discover their food allergies and yeast problems—which are great contributors to distended stomachs—the weight will drop off, so the pressure of all that added weight on the back muscles is greatly reduced.

Elderly people often complain of hip, knee, and joint pain. A lady who came to the clinic was investigating having her knee joints replaced due to severe arthritis. It turned out that she was allergic to *every* food that she was eating. After a period of dietary management and appropriate nutritional supplementation, the pain in her knees was alleviated, and she avoided an expensive and complicated surgical process.

Elaine's Case

Elaine came to me because her teeth were falling out. Often loose teeth stem from a vitamin B deficiency. One of the most beneficial ways for the body to utilize iron and B vitamins, which we all need, is through the consumption of red meat. Red meat has received a bad rap over the years, and Elaine had believed this negative programming. Yet, despite what she'd heard, Elaine began to increase her intake of red meat. Within several weeks, her teeth began to feel more solid in her jaw, and she was spared the loss of more teeth.

No amount of dental work, chiropractic adjustments, or emotional processing would have corrected Elaine's problem. Her body knew what it wanted, and it was going to continue to tell her so with every loose tooth until the message was heard.

What Our Bones May Be Trying to Tell Us

On an emotional level, skeletal systems can be quite revealing. The skeletal structure is the foundation of the body. A weak or imbalanced skeleton may reveal where the structure of your outer life could be chaotic or breaking down. Teeth, in fact, can be linked to areas of pain in the physical body. Did you know that each tooth corresponds energetically to an organ or system in the body? A visit to your holistic dentist can identify which teeth may be compromised or infected—thus contributing to weakened organs and ongoing health problems.

There are ways of looking at painful areas of the body and establishing emotional correlations to them. One of the most popular books on the subject of the connection between emotions and health and disease is *Heal Your Body*, by Louise L. Hay (Hay House, 1984). This book lists every part of the body and the metaphysical reasons for disease in that area. In addition, it provides a positive correlation and affirmative statement to assist in healing each particular body part.

When I work with people, I'll get an intuitive "ding" (or message) about an emotional correlation for skeletal imbalances, and I often receive intuitive associations. For instance, the neck has long been seen, metaphysically, as the division between the head and the heart. Often people with neck pain, or even throat problems, can be experiencing a lack of alignment between what their head is saying to them and what their heart is feeling about a certain subject. As soon as this alignment is corrected, and body toxins are reduced, neck pain usually lessens. Shoulders are related to burden—the person is feeling the weight of the world on their shoulders. Legs and backs are related to support—the legs support the body, and weak legs can't support a body that is unhealthy or emotionally overtaxed. Knees are related to money ("my-knee"), as well as bending to the higher will and surrendering (on our knees) to the Divine in our lives.

Back injuries don't just occur from lifting too much weight or straining the muscles—they're often related to financial or emotional support. The next time your back goes out, look at what might have occurred in your emotional life and where you feel unsupported, or look at possible financial strain.

Feet have to do with understanding—that is, what we're standing on, what our platform is, what we believe in, and how solid we feel in these areas. But I have witnessed many improvements in a person with foot problems when they're supplied with correct nutritional support. Just the avoidance of wheat alone can bring about an improvement in hot, swollen, or tired feet.

The head is related to thinking—usually too much of it. People who are "in their head" would benefit from the peaceful practice of meditation. When the pressure of mental strain is lifted from the body, healing energy moves in to assist in physical well-being. Meditation should be an important part of any health program. (In Chapter 16, I'll give you specific guidelines for meditation that will enhance this tool for optimum health.)

In the quest for ideal health, we need to remember that *anything* that we eat, drink, touch, or breathe can have an adverse effect on every area of our body. In the next chapter, I'll delve into the fascinating topic of the environment—both at home and at work—and show you how your home and work spaces can give you clues to the way you feel.

Chapter 9

Environmental Factors

Due to my background in environmental medicine, I'm very attuned to various environmental factors and their effects on the clients whom I see. People are often surprised to learn that the feathers on their beds, the plants in their bedrooms, or the pets that they love may be contributing to their health problems. Your environment, particularly the one you sleep or work in, requires close scrutiny. Your aim is to create a "safe" place, so take a look at the places where you spend the most amount of your time, and use your intuition to discern any environmental factors that could be disturbing your well-being.

The Home

Sinus congestion, respiratory problems, asthma, puffiness/bags under the eyes, and skin problems are often aggravated by exposures to feathers, dust, molds, chemicals, and pets. Do your best to create an environment where there's little or no contact with these elements, particularly in the bedroom.

The physical components of the bedroom aren't the only ones to consider—where you sleep should be like a healing chamber where you feel supported and protected. After all, you do spend a great deal of time in your bedroom; therefore, you should only be surrounded by items that you love. Choose colors, textures, and fabrics that are pleasant and calming for you. Let the comfort of these surroundings transport you to the deep levels of dreams and rejuvenation.

On a subtle, but very important level, some people have difficulty sleeping because . . . they're sleeping with the wrong person. When you sleep with someone, it's important that your energies match, unite, and merge. There should be such love between you that, in the sleep state, you're bonded like two feathers in the wind, free to soar to the highest realms.

David's Case

I remember when David came to me for a consultation. Among other things, he was having difficulty sleeping. When I mentioned the concept of sleeping with the right person, he was shocked at first, but this theory began to make sense to him because his girlfriend wanted to have a child with him. Although David cared about her, he didn't *love* her. So, when he was close to her in bed, subconsciously he just couldn't override their lack of harmony. David finally started to deeply evaluate this relationship—he needed to have the courage to free the woman he cared about so that she could find the man who would want to become the father of her children . . . and David needed to risk spending time alone in order to find himself.

If you sleep with a feather pillow, you breathe, sweat, and drool into it all night long. This moisture then penetrates the pillow, and various strains of molds can grow among the damp feathers. Night after night, when you put your head on the pillow, the heat from your body warms up the feathers. The molds and dust then rise out of the pillow and come in contact with your nasal passages and respiratory system, thus contributing to puffy eyes or a stuffy nose. Tune in—do you think that your pillow is bothering you? If you have a sensitive respiratory tract or breathing problems, immediately remove feathers from the bed—this includes quilts or duvets.

But don't despair. Take the quilt and pillows off the bed for a few weeks. It's interesting to note that the gastrointestinal tract (guts), lungs, and sinuses are all on the same acupuncture meridian or energy pathway. As your digestive system improves, so will your lungs and sinuses. You may be able to put the feather quilt back on the bed, because quilts usually rest over the shoulders and aren't normally up near the face. But you'll most likely breathe better without the feather pillow, which should be replaced with a synthetic, nonallergenic pillow.

All bedding, including the mattress pad, should be tumbled in a hot clothes dryer for ten minutes, hung out on a clothesline, or aired in the hot sun once a week. The heat will destroy the airborne molds, along with dust particles and mites harbored in the bedding.

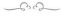

Dust particles and mites abound in bedrooms and also contribute to breathing problems. These tiny particles and microscopic creatures live off the dead skin cells of human beings that are sloughed off in the bedding. Dust mites look huge and grotesque under a magnifying glass. They can contribute to all kinds of problems, such as coughing, itchy and watery eyes, respiratory difficulties, and puffiness and bags under the eyes. It's impossible to get rid of dust mites completely, but it helps to give your entire home and bedroom a thorough cleaning once a week. Remove all extraneous articles and bric-a-brac that could be gathering dust.

I remember visiting friends for dinner one night. After we ate, my friends put on some lively polka music, and several people started dancing around the living room in joyful response. Suddenly, everyone in the room was coughing violently from the dust that rose from the carpet. You could even see the dust particles swirling around in the light. So, if you have a chronic cough, you may want to take a good look at the dust in your environment.

Some people respond to an air purifier in their sleeping areas. I have a silent purifier in my bedroom that filters the air in the room several times an hour; the air always feels crisp and clean. If you're fortunate enough to know a medical doctor or practitioner in your area who specializes in environmental medicine, you can be tested for allergies to dust, molds, feathers, and other airborne inhalants.

Neutralizing drops may give you some relief. The purpose of this kind of treatment is to neutralize or desensitize the body to the effect of each of these allergens—in this way, you can actually tolerate exposure to them without adverse reactions.

Molds

I've mentioned that molds can accumulate in feather pillows and damp bedding, but they're also found in the soil of houseplants. For people with breathing problems, it's wise to remove plants from the bedroom. When they're watered, the molds in their soil can rise into the air and contaminate the space where you're sleeping. The effects from exposure to such molds include breathing problems, puffy eyes, runny noses, postnasal drip, headaches, anxiety, and depression. People who live in damp climates where they are frequently exposed to molds due to rainy weather or dampness are especially prone to these symptoms. During the summer, when the weather is drier, their ailments often improve.

I've seen people's personalities change due to exposure to molds—they can become violent, anxious, or very sad. Several years ago, I visited a farming community where many of the residents were severely affected by molds. All too often these people had musty, damp basements that had been turned into children's playrooms; or computer, sewing, or laundry rooms. I was stunned by the number of people in that community who had environmental illness due to molds. In fact, I met one woman there who finally got relief from her severe migraine headaches when she moved out of her damp dwelling.

While I was in the area, I had the chance to visit an architect at his home. The design of this house was rather interesting, as it bordered a lake and blended with the terrain. But my interest was piqued when the architect led me inside the house. Because I've been trained to detect the smell of mold, my senses were assaulted the moment the front door opened. There were plants trailing everywhere. Beautiful, exotic foliage wound its way through every room in the house. It was hard to get into the dining room due to the number of plants.

As I've said, plants contain molds, which live in the soil. When a plant is watered, mold rises out of the soil and contaminates the immediate environment. If the outside climate in the location is also damp, houseplants and their inherent mold content compound the problem. This poor man I was visiting had breathing problems and was constantly clearing his throat. He had no idea that the plants he loved so much were at the root (no pun intended) of his problems.

❦

Following are two cases relating to cancer and a possible mold connection. Both of these people were subjected to molds in the environment in two different areas of the country. Because molds are so pervasive in damp climates, it's difficult to encourage people to take this issue seriously.

Sonia's Case

Sonia came to me when she was seriously ill with cancer. Nothing short of a miracle would give her the healing she sought. I had little to offer her, save for a few suggestions I intuitively felt might take the pressure off her immune system, allowing it to use its meager reserves in the healing process. Thanks to the rugged lifestyle she was leading, coupled with her exposure to various strains of mold, the pressure on her immune system was very great indeed.

Sonia had suffered many emotional hills and valleys throughout her adult life, and at that time, she and her husband were just barely eking out an existence, living in what resembled a shanty in a small town. The climate was very moldy and damp. As I tuned in to the bedroom area of their home, I got a sinking feeling. It turned out that Sonia and her husband slept on a padded cotton-type mattress in which mold had been accumulating for many years. In addition, there had been a flood in the home their year before and the carpet was never removed, nor had the place been thoroughly dried out. Mold was growing under the carpet, contaminating the environment—and Sonia's breathing passages.

I suggested that Sonia and her husband remove

the mold-ridden bed and carpet, air out the bedroom, and place a dehumidifier in the home. At last report, Sonia's breathing passages had improved, and she slept better in the bedroom than she had in years. Molds, of course, weren't the cause of her problem, but they may have been hampering her recovery.

Reg's Case

Reg contacted me from Pennsylvania, which is well known for its humid summers and damp springs and autumns. He'd had two recurrences of lung cancer. As I tuned in, I knew that his system was laboring. I instinctively felt that it was important to review any of the areas that could be taxing his respiratory tract. In Chinese medicine, the lungs relate to grief, and Reg was grieving the loss of a son who had died tragically in an automobile accident several years before.

We set about cleaning up his environment so that his body would have a chance to fight the cancer. Reg was willing to try anything. I got a sense that his home was contaminated with mold and mildew. When I asked him about the mold content of his home, he admitted that his family had just moved into a rented home that was very dank. I was horrified. At least it was a rented home and another move wasn't an impossible proposition. I suggested that his family consider renting a home away from woods and trees—preferably one that was built high above the ground.

Upon questioning Reg about his diet, I found that it was loaded with sugar and carbohydrates. There's some evidence to show that cancer cells are glucose supported. We also know that candida albicans yeast is a mold, a spore that lives in the body and thrives on starches and sugars. It also flourishes on fermented foods such as beer, wine, mushrooms, pickles, aged cheeses, and fermented condiments—and Reg was quite a beer drinker.

Candida albicans yeast lives on all the mucous membranes of the human body—namely the lungs, where dark, moist passages offer it a welcome home. Reg was battling mold on the inside, as well as on the outside. A candida albicans yeast-eradication program, along with a major reduction in sugars and ferments, have brought him some relief. His family also moved to a drier location. Molds weren't the reason for Reg's weakened state; however, when his body was helped by the removal of negative environmental factors, there was a greater chance for healing.

Investigate the possibilities of molds in your home. For instance, clean up and dry out your basement. If your home is slightly moldy and damp, purchase a dehumidifier, which will help remove the moisture in the air. Never allow a child to sleep (or yourself to work) in such a place. Go into these places with the nose of a bloodhound, and use your instincts to correct problems. If you suspect that your home is moldy, and you have a child or family member who suffers from anxiety or depression, there may be a connection.

If you currently live in a moist place, limit the intake of mold from your food. Avoid eating mushrooms, vinegar, pickles, soy sauce, aged cheeses, wine, and beer—which are all fermented items—until your mold sensitivities subside. After you've avoided these items for approximately 30 days, reintroduce these items and watch for symptoms. Is your nose runny? Do you feel the onset of a headache? During this whole process—in which you're developing your intuition—use your own body as a laboratory to see the effects of the environment on your system.

(Incidentally, if you're purchasing a home or an apartment, look for a dwelling that's built well above the ground, has good air circulation, and comes with a dry basement or crawl space.)

Our Fine Furry (and Feathered) Friends

As adorable and precious as pets are, they're also the breeding grounds for some not-so-adorable parasites, worms, bacteria, and infectious strains of disease. Animal hair and dander can also be highly allergic for some people, especially those suffering from respiratory problems and asthma. Many people sleep with cats, dogs, ferrets, rodents, and even snakes!

Treya's Case

Treya was a pet owner who had been suffering from asthma for many years. She used an inhaler several times a day and was unable to participate in any strenuous activity for fear of triggering an asthma attack. Respiratory tract infections can be greatly helped by the elimination of milk and dairy products, so Treya removed these items from her diet immediately and her condition began to improve.

The next step was to change her living environment—especially the bedroom. Treya lived in a dry area of the country, so the addition of a humidifier to counteract the dry climate was a positive benefit.

Several months later, Treya called to say that she

had improved greatly and only needed to use her inhaler approximately three times a week. But I intuited that her four cats were the last remaining part of the problem, and Treya didn't want to remove them from the house.

A year later, Treya called to say that she'd finally made a decision that worked for her—the cats were happy living in the garage, and her children enjoyed playing with them outdoors. All the carpet in the home had been replaced with tile to remove any traces of cat hair and dander. She was delighted to report that the inhaler was "a thing of the past," and for the first time in her life, she was enjoying hiking, basketball, and other vigorous exercise.

Parasites can be another problem when it comes to cats and dogs. I don't mean to be graphic, but these furry, lovable creatures are sleeping on your bed and sitting on your pillow after they've spent the day roaming around in the world. They've been having a lovely time, sniffing other creatures' bottoms and genitalia, along with fire hydrants and convenient bushes, in search of any scent that attracts them. Then they return home to lick your face and hands and sit on the pillow that you'll lay your head on at night.

Intuitively, I often pick up the feeling that parasites are present in many people, especially children. Due to poor personal hygiene, children can often be wonderful hosts for parasites. Such children may appear pale, listless, whiny, or agitated; may be scratching themselves; and may be unable to sit still. Quite often, they have pinworms, which are easily transmitted and easily eradicated. Teach your children about parasites and how they're transmitted. It may not always be the best thing to have a pet lick a child on the mouth. Teach children to wash their hands after touching pets, and always before handling food.

If you own pets, research information about natural remedies for parasites, and administer them to your family twice a year. Or ask your doctor to examine and test your children for parasites. Also, be sure that your pet has had up-to-date shots, has been frequently dewormed, and gets regular veterinary attention.

Vivian's Case

Vivian called me a number of years ago, suffering from fatigue. As I spoke to her, the thought came to my mind that she might have been dealing with intestinal parasites. I asked her if she had a cat—she didn't, but she did have birds. I figured that the birds would be in a cage, and Vivian was just handling the birds without washing her hands. Wrong. *About 30 birds were flying free all over Vivian's house.* They were landing and pooping on her kitchen counters, as well as perching on the kitchen dishcloth that was conveniently draped over the faucet.

The dishcloth was used to wipe the counters before Vivian prepared her meals and washed her dishes afterwards. This was an interesting scenario, and an easy way for parasites, which almost every animal carries, to enter into Vivian's body and contaminate her system. The remedy was simple—contain the birds and take a short course of an anti-parasitic botanical to eliminate the parasites and their eggs. Shortly after this treatment, Vivian's energy returned.

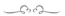

Many people maintain very poor standards of cleanliness. I'm often horrified to hear that people use the same cloth to wipe the floor and counters that they use to clean their baby's face! Kitchen cloths and sponges are loaded with germs and bacteria and should be washed or bleached on a daily basis. Every day, a clean dishcloth should replace the one from the day before.

Since I grew up in a medical family, my father actually used to inspect the dishes every night while we children were washing them. This was long before the days of dishwashers. He would often take a glass of rinse water, hold it up to the light, and ask us pointedly, "Can you drink this?" In our household, the rinse water had to be hot and pristine—even when we went camping, which we did as a family quite often. Those trips were always fun, but I can still smell the disinfectant that my parents would liberally pour into every bucket of dishwater and each hand-washing basin. So it was with our medical family. I'm not suggesting that you have to take such extreme steps, but do pay close attention to germs and personal hygiene.

Chemical Sensitivities

Many people react adversely to chemicals. When people have weakened immune systems and are plagued with the candida yeast syndrome (which further weakens the immune system), they can find themselves chemically sensitive. The most common culprits are tobacco smoke, scents and perfumes, cleaning compounds, and gasoline fumes—formaldehyde and chlorine can also cause reactions in some people. Often new building materials, floor coverings, and paints are extremely toxic.

Take, for example, a CNS stress person. These people give their power away and characteristically have weak or reactive immune systems. They will often react to perfume—

feeling nervous, high-strung, or headachey when they're exposed to the perfumes that they spray on themselves. This is because they don't have the reserves in their immune system "bank account" to handle the assault of the perfume, nail polish, scent, or any other chemical that pervades their personal environment. If you're a CNS type and want to wear perfume, look for essential oils, which are made from natural plant extracts. However, many people can even react to these scents because they can be yet another element for a sensitive immune system to handle.

Cleaning solutions, which are highly pungent, can also compound the problem. Strongly scented laundry soaps, for instance, can contribute to breathing problems or skin irritations. Choose unscented laundry detergents and cleaning compounds, which can be found at your local health-food store.

A client of mine, Diana, had a persistent raspy cough. We isolated her food allergies, removed her cat from the bedroom, and exchanged her down pillow for a hypoallergenic one. Diana's cough subsided, but it didn't disappear completely. Upon further investigation, it was discovered that Diana used a laundry detergent with an intense scent, and her clothing and bedding continually emitted this fragrance. She began using an unscented detergent and her cough cleared up.

The Office

Many people who work in large buildings with central heating and air-conditioning systems can be affected with what's known as *toxic building syndrome*. The air that they're breathing may not have been properly circulated or purified, and consequently, they're deprived of good-quality air. They can also be impacted by those ever-present fluorescent lights. It's no wonder that more and more people are choosing to work from home, where they can open windows and control the quality of the air they breathe.

If you do find yourself in one of these large office buildings, ask the maintenance manager to examine the air filters to ensure that they're frequently cleaned and that the air is circulating properly. Bring in a small desktop air purifier, which will enhance the quality of the air in your personal work space.

Remember to take frequent breaks outside: for every two hours of work, a five-minute fresh-air break should be taken. Strengthen your immune system with nutritional supplementation to support your body. Watch your intake of caffeine and sugars, which are an assault on your adrenal glands (your fight-or-flight mechanism) and will ultimately tire your system. Eat healthful foods—do your best to avoid pastries and muffins that give you a temporary boost in energy but then plummet you downward into a low-blood-sugar spiral. And last, but not least—choose jobs and careers where the environment is as supportive as possible—on all levels.

Electromagnetic Stress

The human body is surrounded by a delicately balanced electromagnetic system, also known as the *aura*. Every living thing has this electromagnetic field or aura around it. When you're receptive and open to seeing on this level, you can see the aura around any living thing—animals, human beings, trees, flowers, and plants. This is the radiation of the life force around the living thing, which is necessary for its protection, and a very vital part of its system. I'm fortunate to be able to see auras, which isn't difficult—it takes training and receptivity, and then it becomes obvious. Once you begin to see the aura around every living thing, you can never go back to just looking at a person, a tree, or a flower in the same way.

Current research and information shows that there may be some concern regarding electromagnetic frequencies and their effect on the body and the protective aura that surrounds it. Microwaves, cell phones, computers, high-tension wires, and electromagnetic influences of all kinds may impact the protection of our own subtle electromagnetic field. When I was an allergy tester, electromagnetic stress would regularly show up when I tested sick people. Quite simply, it's another stress on the system that the body has to cope with.

Many elderly, frail, or ill people have very narrow or fragile auras because their electromagnetic systems are ultrasensitive. Therefore, electromagnetic influences such as heating pads and electric blankets can interfere with the delicate balance of their electromagnetic systems, especially if they're CNS types.

Picture an elderly lady wearing a nylon nightgown. The static electricity created by her nightgown, along with the polyester sheets she uses, can disturb the subtle electromagnetic field around her body. Then imagine that she climbs into bed and covers herself with an electric blanket, which further disrupts her delicate electromagnetic field. The effects of these elements can charge or overcharge the nervous system, possibly disturbing sleep, balance, physical health, and emotional well-being.

In order to avoid undue electromagnetic stress on your body, wear cotton or natural fibers next to your skin. Sleep between 100 percent cotton sheets, and use an old-fashioned hot-water bottle for warmth in order to avoid undue exposure to electrical influences near the body. Seek help in testing your home environment for high levels of electromagnetic stress, and research useful devices to protect yourself from such interference.

Molly's Case

This story goes back to my clinical days. Ten-year-old Molly had leukemia, and she was so pale and weak that you could almost see right through her. It turned out that she had a major milk allergy—and her parents owned a dairy. She also showed up positive on the testing for electromagnetic stress, which determines the effects of electromagnetic influences on the body.

When people are weak and sick, these electric frequencies can have an adverse effect. Upon inquiry, Molly's parents said that there was an electronic substation right outside her bedroom window, which provided the power for their home, the dairy, and surrounding buildings. When the doctor discussed the possibility of moving the family to another location due to the potential this amount of electricity presented to a very sick little girl, Molly's distraught mother cried, "But this is my dream home." Some dream!

Seasonal Affective Disorder

As soon as autumn sets in, numerous people become depressed or suffer from low moods and energy due to the lack of natural light. This "sunlight shortage" affects one of the major endocrine glands, the pineal gland. This gland, located in the head, is involved in hormone function, as well as energy and mood regulation. The depression felt when the pineal gland is starving for light is called seasonal affective disorder, or SAD. Unfortunately, this syndrome isn't well recognized, and when it *is* diagnosed, the treatments are usually complicated, time-consuming, and expensive.

Many years ago, however, a skilled group of alternative

practitioners that I know discovered an inexpensive way of treating SAD: Take an ordinary pocket flashlight with you when you go to bed at night, turn it on, and hold it to the center of your forehead for about three minutes. This process effectively floods your brain cavity with powerful light. Repeat this simple procedure every night before sleeping and every morning upon waking for approximately three weeks, and then once or twice a week after that. It won't take long before you'll notice an improvement in energy and mood.

Environmental Illness

When I was an allergy-testing technician, I had a chance to see many people with environmental illness. These people suffered from poor-quality air, chemical sensitivities, multiple food allergies, airborne pollutants, and so on. These were some very distressed people.

Environmental illness is difficult to treat. Like an onion, you have to start at the beginning and peel back the layers to get at its core. I usually begin by isolating food allergies. The next steps are to remove toxic substances from the environment, support the body with correct supplementation, use desensitizing drops to neutralize the patient for elements in the environment, and most important, dig out the buried emotion or stress that's weakening the system in the first place. Environmentally ill people often have emotional baggage that lies buried beneath the surface.

Gretchen's Case

Gretchen was in her mid-30s when she was admitted to the clinic. She was so environmentally ill that she used a gas mask in order to breathe. It turned out that as a child, she'd frequently been severely beaten and locked in a closet; and as an added punishment, she was often deprived of food. Gretchen's body just couldn't thrive under the onslaught of the emotional trauma she'd endured. Over the years, her body got weaker and weaker, to the point that it eventually broke down and she became what is termed a *universal reactor*. She reacted to everything in the environment. The object of environmental medicine is to establish and remove these factors—in Gretchen's case, there were many.

Expert complementary medical attention and deep emotional work have given Gretchen a chance to experience life as it's supposed to be lived. Many years have passed, and she's now a complementary medical practitioner herself and enjoying excellent health.

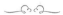

Not everyone who suffers from environmental illness has emotional issues. Perfectly well-adjusted people can be severely afflicted by exposure to toxic wastes, heavy metal absorption, poisoned water, natural gas leaks, and chemical emissions. These are isolated cases, and each one is handled individually with competent medical attention. If people are healthy to begin with, they'll eventually recover from these exposures.

If you're experiencing symptoms, look at your personal environment with the eye of a detective. The key to handling a toxic environment is a healthy immune system. As our world and our immediate environment become more and more populated, toxic, and polluted, the answer lies (apart from advocacy) in maintaining a strong body with which to cope with them.

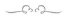

In Part III, I'll introduce you to some of the interesting cases I've worked on over the years. I hope that from these revealing insights, you'll observe how a medical intuitive interacts with people and how you can gain greater understanding about some of the components involved in your health issues.

PART III

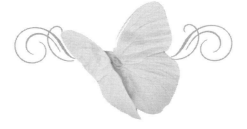

Special Cases

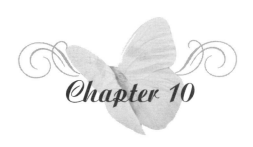

Chapter 10

Simple Body Imbalances

Each body's physical system reacts differently, demonstrating its own unique capacity to respond to simple changes in dramatic or subtle ways. I look for visual signs of imbalance and use inner vision to "see" into organs and systems. The body tells me what it wants. I visualize each person in a state of health and wellness, for I believe that this actually shifts the energy and propels them in that direction. I stay attuned to my inner voice and "knowing," and my specific background and training acts as a filter for the data I get. I receive my impressions very quickly—all of the perceptions I receive seem to "bank up" above and around my head, and I need to stay focused as I "pull" each one of them down. I'm continually scanning the body and "combing" through the information that I'm given, since this download of material is random and unsorted. After the data is disseminated, and there's no further information seemingly "hanging" in space, I know that this intense and rapid-fire process is complete. I then formulate my impressions into a practical framework, which I subsequently write down and discuss with the client.

The following case histories illustrate how medical

intuitive impressions come to me on the physical, emotional, or spiritual planes, and how these individuals may have benefited from some of my suggestions. The body's capacity to regenerate is phenomenal—just the removal of some common substances can bring about dramatic changes.

Linda's Case

Several years ago, I was invited to speak at a health conference. While I was there, I consulted with Linda, who told me she had 30 benign breast cysts. She had to endure a painful procedure as each cyst was excised—which consisted of inserting a needle into the cyst to draw out the fluid. Even though her case seemed rather complicated, my impression was that she should simply stop drinking coffee and eating dairy products for a short period of time. This would take the pressure off her lymphatic system, allowing it to drain.

Linda's main imbalances were in her digestive, lymphatic, and endocrine systems. Dairy products and caffeine can often block the lymphatic system, contributing to lumps or cysts, not to mention related premenstrual syndrome (PMS) symptoms. Sometimes just the avoidance of dairy and caffeine can bring relief.

After four weeks, Linda called to say that, thankfully, she only had three cysts left, and they were shrinking. As an additional benefit, she was delighted to report that she hadn't been subjected to her usual PMS-related maladies. The body is remarkable. It knows just what to do if it's given a chance.

—ℰ⌒ℰ⌒—

In my medical intuitive work, I notice that many people who consume caffeine have anger and irritation just below the surface, not to mention various physical problems. Several years ago, a study was done by the National Aeronautics and Space Administration (NASA) regarding the effects of caffeine and other mood-altering substances on spiders and their web-weaving techniques. Webs constructed when the spiders were exposed to caffeine appeared as a loose, haphazard array of crooked and incomplete spokes. The spiders were unable to perform their natural functions in an organized manner while under the influence of such a stimulant.

It's the same with sensitive human beings. Imagine all of the people that you know who perform delicate and important functions in top-level professions—and who rely upon copious amounts of caffeine to stay alert. People often blame their life circumstances for the way they feel when they actually need to look closely at their stimulant intake. Not only can caffeine contribute to emotional instability, it can also increase the heart rate or elevate blood pressure.

Take Ed for instance. He was a 45-year-old man we worked with in the naturopathic clinic. Ed said he drank 15 cups of coffee a day and also had other food allergies. On that first visit, we just asked him to eliminate coffee. Six weeks later, he arrived at the clinic to tell us that he was no longer yelling at his children, his relationship with his wife was much better, and he was relating to his co-workers in a more positive manner—and all of this was because he stopped ingesting caffeine.

Special Imbalances in Children and Young Adults

Babies can often inherit their parents' allergic tendencies. Janet and her son were perfect examples of this.

Janet's Case

Janet was distraught because her infant son had recurrent respiratory and ear infections. In his short life, he'd required several courses of antibiotics. He constantly cried and rubbed his ears, and Janet frequently had to sit up with him all night just so he could breathe more easily—but she was mystified as to how to alleviate his pain.

Janet was breast-feeding her baby son, and hadn't realized that this was a problem—she was passing her own allergies along to her baby.

I'd already done several consultations for this family, so I knew that Janet's husband and five-year-old son, as well as Janet herself, were highly allergic to dairy. In fact, whenever Janet drank milk or ate dairy products, she felt puffy and retained fluid. Consequently, she had difficulty maintaining normal body weight.

But nursing mothers are usually *supposed* to drink a good supply of milk each day—isn't milk supposed to supply calcium and other important nutrients to mothers and newborn infants? Not so in every case. This particular mother was highly milk-allergic, and so was her baby—he inherited this allergy genetically, and it was also transmitted through Janet's breast milk.

Since the child had been on so many courses of antibiotics, which can disturb the delicate balance of intestinal flora, I started by suggesting that a bowel bacteria culture might be useful in returning this area to normal. My main piece of advice, however, was to eliminate milk from both Janet's diet and that of her son. Immediately after Janet stopped drinking milk, her son could breathe more easily, and after a few days, his ears were less inflamed. "It happened so fast, it was like a miracle," Janet told me.

Robert's Case

Nine-year-old Robert and his distraught mother came to me for a consultation. Robert had been diagnosed with mild autism—autistic children can often appear absent, incommunicative, and engage in repeated behavior patterns. The mother was beside herself trying to control this boy who couldn't be left alone for a moment without a resulting calamity. When I looked at Robert, I could see that he was "in there"—that is, within himself, he was "home," or present and aware of his surroundings. He didn't appear to have the usual signs of autism. I preferred to see him intuitively as a small boy with behavior problems, food allergies, and chemical imbalances. Because the only way Robert's mother could handle her son was to give him whatever he wanted, he ate and drank anything he pleased.

I suggested to the mother that she implement a ten-day "clear" program, so the foods and beverages Robert was allergic to, and to which he was constantly exposed, wouldn't be consumed.

After ten days, the mother contacted me to say that this was the first time she'd had any peace since Robert was born. His mood swings were predictable and less severe, and he was calmer and happier with himself and his surroundings. Even his teachers commented on the change in him. Over time, his mother became acutely aware of dramatic shifts in his behavior when he consumed dairy products, preservatives, food dyes, or sugars—and that exposure just wasn't worth the price of family disruption. At last report, Robert continues to progress.

Greg's Case

Greg, a teenager, was pale and lethargic. Using my intuitive eyes, I looked into his intestinal tract and could see that it was angry and irritated. It turned out that he'd been battling an inflammatory condition of the bowels—consequently, he'd been suffering from cramps and diarrhea and weighed less than 80 pounds. At the same time, he had a history of antibiotic treatment due to repeated respiratory infections. Greg was also plagued with recurring bladder infections. Bladder and yeast infections are related symptoms of chronic candidiasis. This boy was consuming vast amounts of sugar, soda pop, and fruit juice, and as I've said, candida thrives on sugars in any form.

We set about to reduce his sugar consumption, and I suggested some foods that might be less irritating to his colon. He'd been everywhere to find relief, but I felt that it was important for him to see a holistic physician and begin treatment for candidiasis. Within three weeks, Greg's cramps and diarrhea had stopped, and he was feeling stronger and more energetic than ever. A month later, he'd gained five pounds, and was doing better than he had in a very long time.

Arthritis and Joint Disorders

Afflictions of the joints, including arthritis, are almost accepted as inevitable signs of aging. This doesn't have to be so, as the following cases will illustrate.

Ruby's Case

Ruby came to me with a history of rheumatoid arthritis attacks. This painful disease involves the body's immune system, which actually attacks itself. Many times, Ruby's symptoms were so severe that she had to be hospitalized, and she was treated with strong drugs to keep her condition at bay. After a ten-year remission, her symptoms flared up again, and this is when I saw her. Ruby was pale and exhausted, and her pain was so severe that she was unable to walk, which was extremely stressful for her, considering that she made her living as a waitress. Several vials of fluid were surgically removed from her knees due to pressure buildup. She was one of The Tricky People, but I tried to help her anyway.

Looking at Ruby, I could tell that she was allergic to grains. Glutinous grains can often contribute to joint pain, both mild and severe. Onions and garlic were also factors, as these frequently consumed foods can contribute to digestive problems and immune reactions in some people. In addition, Ruby appeared sensitive to the *nightshade food family* (see Food Family list on page 277), which is comprised of potatoes, tomatoes, eggplant, tobacco, and peppers in any form. The nightshade family may be linked to arthritis, although this sensitivity rarely showed up in my work as an allergy tester. And last, I detected that unmistakable yeasty smell wafting through the room—it seemed as if candida yeast was at it again.

I suggested that Ruby eliminate grains and foods in the nightshade family, and work to eliminate candida. Within three days of following her plan, her agony was noticeably diminished. After a week, the pain and swelling had almost disappeared completely. Two weeks later, she was back at work and no longer suffering. Ruby continued on a candida-erad-ication program for several months, and was careful to monitor her offending foods, keeping exposure to a minimum.

In reviewing this case, I found that the core ele-ment in Ruby's condition was the dissatisfaction she felt as a waitress. She'd been disregarding her creative abilities and putting stress on her body and immune system with such demanding physical work. Exam-ining why she was waiting tables instead of waiting *on herself* and bringing forth the gifts that she had to offer the world assisted her in addressing the emo-tional nature of her illness. Once Ruby confronted these issues and followed the right food plan, she ultimately was able to heal.

Dennis's Case

Dennis came to me with severe joint pain. He loved to go ballroom dancing but had given it up due to his condition. No amount of supplements or pain relievers seemed to be working. I tuned in and quickly discerned that the elimination of wheat would help him. He consumed vast amounts of pasta, which is made from wheat flour. When peo-ple are sensitive to wheat and other glutinous grains, they can often have joint problems due to an immune reaction and resulting inflammation. I also suggested that he take sugar—a major culprit—out of his diet for the same 30-day trial period.

After a month, Dennis reported back to me to say that he was back to ballroom dancing and was even doing deep knee bends. He was free of pain, and his body was responding to the new regime of meals with rice or potatoes, instead of pasta.

In reviewing this case, I found out that Dennis had suffered profound losses in his life, which had affected his body, particularly his immune system. The immune system can become compromised and reactive when people suffer from emotional upheavals. Dennis had been divorced three times—at great emotional and financial expense—thus putting additional strain on his organs and joints. As I've previously mentioned, knees, on an emotional level, can relate to money, flexibility, and surrendering to the higher will or to the greater picture. Once Dennis acknowledged his emotional obstacles, and also followed the proper food plan, he was well on the road to recovery.

In the next chapter, I'll show you how a particular lifestyle choice can affect the subtle balance of physical well-being, and how medical intuition can assist in unraveling some obvious physical symptoms that go hand-in-hand with this way of life.

Chapter 11

Vegetarianism and Your Health

For the past 20 years, there has been a great interest in vegetarianism due to the use of hormones and antibiotics in meat, along with the reported inhumane treatment of animals being slaughtered. Many people are concerned about these important issues, and justifiably so. I don't want to get into politics here—I just want to discuss the direct effects of the vegetarian lifestyle on one's health. I've had such a long history of working with so many types of people in a clinical setting that I've had the chance to observe countless vegetarians.

Vegetarians were among the sickest people that we treated during my clinical days due to their sensitive gastrointestinal tracts and predilections for high-starch and/or high-sugar diets. It was ironic that these people, who only strived for vibrant health, were often actually quite ill.

In my experience as a medical intuitive, I've noticed that CNS types, whose main problem involves handling sugar, don't do well on a vegetarian diet, since almost everything they're eating is either sugar to begin with, or rapidly becomes sugar in the digestive process.

DLH types, however, appear to respond more favorably

to a diet of vegetables, whole grains, and legumes—especially if they're of Asian or African-American extraction.

Sensitive digestive systems and emotions—along with a lack of absorbable protein, iron, and B vitamins—seem to play a key role in the success or failure of a vegetarian plan. In fact, the "m" word in my vocabulary doesn't stand for marriage or menopause, it stands for *meat*—our consumption of which has been declining over the years as we try to get "healthy" on a low-fat, high-carbohydrate diet! While there are certainly plenty of healthy vegetarians around the world, the following stories illustrate how a vegetarian regimen may not be the best plan for every body.

Catherine's Case

Catherine had been a strict vegetarian for 15 years and had resisted the "m" word. She had *sworn to a guru* that she wouldn't kill an animal to feed herself. When I looked at this woman, I could see that she was way out of balance emotionally. Catherine was a typical CNS type—she was wired and maxed out in all areas. I intuited that she gave her power away and deferred to anyone whom she thought was more important than she was. She experienced such hills and valleys of emotion that much of the time she felt as if she were on a roller coaster. Beyond that, I could see that Catherine was very sensitive, fragile, and absolutely beautiful—both inside and out—just like a delicate, untainted flower.

Looking at her background, I could see that she'd picked up her patterns from her mother, who, despite being a professional woman, gave her power away to others and allowed people to take advantage of her in business and in her personal life. Catherine's mother chose to put up with this kind of treatment because she abhorred confrontation and didn't want to hurt anyone. Catherine had learned this behavior well, and she was following right in her mother's footsteps. She eventually removed herself from mainstream society and was embraced by a "spiritual" community, where she gave her own power and authority over to a guru who decided what was best for her body.

I saw Catherine several years later, and she was a physical and emotional wreck. As I said, she was a CNS person, and this type usually has difficulty managing sugar. A typical vegetarian diet, unless it's well managed, tends to consist mainly of starches and sugar. Because starches convert to sugar in the body, all of that sweetness circulating around in the bloodstream can contribute to a person feeling emotionally unstable. In addition, vegetarians often have multiple food allergies and sensitivities, as well as touchy digestive systems.

I suggested that Catherine add more useful and digestible protein into her diet. Her body wasn't handling or processing beans very well because she had such a fragile digestive system. Many vegetarians, in fact, don't tolerate beans well at all—and they're the mainstay of a vegetarian diet.

We needed to add protein back into her diet, and the "m" word was the only solution. I suggested that we start with fish and chicken. Catherine was aghast to think that she'd have to kill an animal in order to survive. But *everything is killed*. People who "see" these things tell me that even a carrot screams when it's pulled out of the ground—after all, plants have to die so that we can eat them. And in order for the farmer to harvest the grain in his fields or the vegetables in his plots, animal habitats are often destroyed. Native creatures are driven from their homes or nests—after which, they subsequently die. The food chain in the animal world doesn't follow our rules. Wolves kill deer, cougars slay wolves, and certain kinds of snakes in Africa prey on goats and even small children—these animals give no thought to philosophy or consciousness. It's about survival.

I encouraged Catherine to add animal protein into her diet for the next month and observe any changes. Although it wasn't easy for her to make this switch, she reported four weeks later that she felt much more stable on all levels. Due to this increased physical stability, she was able to discern where she needed to hold her power and confidence in relationships; she also realized how much she'd been deferring to others, especially people she felt had all the answers.

At last report, Catherine was thriving.

Donna's Case

Donna came to me with psoriasis patches as big as dinner plates all over her body, which she'd had for more than 20 years. She was also a vegetarian. Unfortunately, Donna's diet was composed mainly of starches and sugar in all forms, which, as we know, candida albicans feeds on. Psoriasis is one of the common symptoms of the candida yeast syndrome—in fact, skin conditions very often result from internal, not external, factors. All the treatment in the world on the outside, or surface of the skin, rarely remedies the problem. But if the correction takes place internally, skin manifestations usually do clear up. (Exceptions are heat rashes, poison oak, insect bites, or other afflictions that *do* take place on the surface of the skin.)

Donna decided to try eating animal protein, along with lots of vegetables and a limited amount of starches. She also took a specific antifungal agent to eradicate her candidiasis. No sugar was the order of the day—even fruit and fruit juices had to go, as they're also sugar! It took a while—several months on a fairly strict regime—but her psoriasis patches have healed, and Donna can now wear shorts and sleeveless dresses.

Ellen's Case

When Ellen came to me for a consultation, she was a competitive gymnast. Despite only being 18 years old, she was experiencing joint pain and was concerned that she wouldn't be able to compete in state gymnastic competitions. Ellen was a vegetarian and was adamant that she wouldn't consume the "m" word.

As I looked at her food allergies, I noticed that she had sensitivities to dairy products and sugar. Thankfully, she did have a healthy stomach and digestive system and wasn't sensitive to beans (legumes). So, the plan was to remove dairy products and sugar in all forms—including honey, fruit juices, and dried fruits (known as "healthy sugars")—from her diet for 30 days. I suggested that she eat heartily from vegetables, some fruits; and as many nuts, beans, and soy products as she wished at every meal. Ellen was fortunate in that she didn't have any sensitivities to grains, so she continued to consume them. At the same time, I suggested an antifungal agent to assist in eradicating candidiasis, which, as I've said, is particularly common among vegetarians due to their high consumption of starches and sugar.

A month later, Ellen reported that her joint inflammation had improved, and she was pain free and able to compete. What's interesting is that the element of perfection required in gymnastics was actually at the root of her discomfort. The exacting nature of this sport had placed added stress on her immune system. So by eliminating offending foods, the additional pressure was taken off her immune system, and Ellen's body was given the chance to heal.

Often, after a period of avoidance to give the digestive tract a chance to repair, vegetarians are able to add soy and assorted legumes back into their diet. The easiest beans to digest are lentils, which are available in a wide variety. Sometimes just adding digestive enzymes assists in the body being able to assimilate beans as usable sources of protein.

Due to a number of multilayered factors, the body can occasionally break down almost beyond its capacity to recover. The next set of cases will show you how I work intuitively with people who are seriously or chronically ill.

Chapter 12

Serious Illnesses

Early in my career, I had the good fortune to work with a doctor who refused to label diseases. "Cancer," he told me, "is just a name. It's the body calling out for help, and our role is to find out what it wants."

For instance, it may be worthwhile to keep in mind that scientists have known for years that most types of cancer cells are "sugar junkies." These fast-growing cells depend on glucose to live. For example, one Johns Hopkins University study found that when cancer cells were denied glucose, they died. Very often, if you examine the diet of someone with cancer, you'll find an overconsumption of sugars and starches in all forms. Tuning in to your body—and nutritional habits—is always a good place to start if you're fighting a serious illness.

If you've been diagnosed with cancer, or any disease, remember that *it's just a label.* Your body is out of balance and most likely knows what to do to repair itself. Open your eyes and your mind, and study and embrace all forms of treatment available to you, both conventional and alternative. Because the mind is so powerful, your *belief* in the forms of treatment that you choose will greatly determine the results you get. But use your common sense, too. Don't hang on to a body part just to prove a point—if it needs to be removed, remove it.

I never label disease; in fact, I prefer not to know anything about the person I'm working with. I like to look at the systems that are out of balance and ask the question, "What does this body want?" Serious illnesses, including cancer, have the capacity to turn around. Here are some interesting cases.

Betsy's Case

Betsy attended one of my group assessments. She was extremely ill; in fact, someone literally carried her into the presentation. I had a fit—who was this person to assume that I'd be able to provide even a shred of assistance for this poor woman?

I took a moment out from the presentation and went over to speak to Betsy privately. I saw a woman who was in substantial pain, and who was very weak and toxic—almost as if the poisons in her body were circulating around inside of her and going nowhere. At this point, I didn't know that she was suffering from breast cancer. As I said, I've learned not to label disease. I stayed quiet so that my instincts could speak to me, and then I asked her friend to grab paper and a pen to write some things down.

The operant word for cancer, like any other labeled, serious illness, is *precious*. When a person's body is in a weakened state, it must be treated as precious. The visual image relating to such a person is a tiny baby bird, fallen from its nest and shivering on the ground below. The bird is lodged in a crack, and there are a few leaves covering it, but it has no nest or mother. However, the sun is shining, and from where the bird is lying, it can look up and see the blue sky. There's hope. So it is with a person fighting a serious illness. If they're treated with gentleness, recovery is possible.

The thought came to me that Betsy needed soup and lots of it. One of the traditional alternative treatments for cancer patients is raw vegetables, which can be useful for some people. Yet many times, sick people have weak digestive systems, and raw foods don't break down well. Such people are also often encouraged to take massive amounts of supplements, which can be difficult to digest as well. I certainly would not call these treatments "precious" for an ill person. Soup, however, is both healing and nurturing. You probably remember your mother giving you soup when you felt under the weather as a small child.

A person with cancer needs to have supportive nutrition, which is highly absorbable and will strengthen the body as it copes with illness. Specific soups are frequently given to me intuitively as part of the healing equation. So I suggested that Betsy have six cups of beef broth per day, as well as several cups of a special South American medicinal tea, which can be helpful for people suffering from cancer. (For more information on this tea, please go to my website: **www.carolinesutherland.com**. My recipe for beef broth can be found on page 266 in "A Basic Food Plan.") We also went over some other dietary changes, such as eliminating sugars, caffeine, and dairy products from her diet—all of which can be a burden to the system. Then Betsy was helped out of the room.

Five months later, I returned to the same city to teach a class in medical intuition. Betsy pulled up in the parking lot, jumped out of her car, threw her arms around me, and started to cry. "You saved my life," she said. Here's her story.

> The day after Caroline's presentation, I was lying on the couch, where I'd spent most of my time for so many months. I was completely debilitated following chemotherapy and the radiation that had badly damaged my lung. When my breast cancer was first discovered, I was given less than three months to live, due to the rate it was moving. I was now recovering at home, barely surviving on vegetable juices, and feeling as if I was going nowhere.

> I thought about what Caroline had suggested the night before. I forced myself to get up and make the beef broth. I was so weak I could hardly stand. While I knew I didn't have any beef bones on hand, I looked in the freezer to discover a small roast of beef, which I placed in the oven. Something made me look in the pantry, and by some miracle, I found the medicinal tea, which I'd purchased the year before on someone's recommendation. I brewed a batch of tea, and as soon as I started drinking it, the soreness in my throat—which had been so painful I couldn't swallow—seemed to back off. The tea felt good and nurturing as it went down into my system, and it seemed to be getting to places in my body that really needed help. The effect was immediate: Two hours later, after I'd consumed several cups of tea and beef broth, I started getting my strength back. I got up, cleaned the house, and made dinner for my family—something they couldn't remember me doing in a very long time.

Two months after following this program, I went to see my doctor for a checkup. All but one of my tumor tags (cancer markers) had returned to normal. The only marker that remained in the high range—it was still normal, but not great—was the metastatic tag, the indicator for the possible recurrence of cancer. It was time to do some more work.

After some intense psychotherapeutic and emotional work, a strict diet, and nutritional support, I received the news that this time my metastatic tag was indeed normal.

I truthfully feel that I wasn't getting anywhere following my conventional cancer treatment. No one could pinpoint the nutritional needs of my body. The question "What does this body want?" hadn't been posed. Now, thanks to all of the approaches that I've followed, both traditional and nontraditional, and all of the people that God has put in my path, I have strength in my body. I'm hiking, I'm riding horses—I have a life.

When I look at Betsy's case, I understand that belief played a key role in her recovery. She *believed* that these practical suggestions would be beneficial—they made sense to her.

As an interesting side note, on an emotional level, breast cancer involves self-love and self-nurturing. The breasts cover or protect the heart, and if we look underneath the breasts to the heart, very often there can be an emotional wound that hasn't healed. In Betsy's case, the "hole in her heart" revolved around her relationship with her husband, which had undergone a particularly difficult period prior to the discovery of her cancer. If you have breast cancer, you need to ask yourself the question:

"Am I taking care of others more than I am nurturing myself?" You may be surprised by the answer that comes to you, but remember—your body always "knows."

Arnold's Case

I met Arnold at one of my seminars. He had a tired, cloudy look about him, and was recovering from a brain tumor. He'd been actively involved as a commodities broker—which meant he was always living in his head. Although he'd taken a leave of absence from his job, and his will to live was evident, he was still lacking something to get him going down the road to a full recovery.

I maintained silence while I listened for inner guidance and direction. I got the strong impression that nature would have a healing effect on him, and I asked Arnold if he had a favorite spot that he liked to visit. "Oh, yes," he answered. "My aunt owns a vineyard, and when I can, I help her with the grapevines. I always feel good there."

Along with the correct diet and nutritional elements, I had the strong impression that Arnold needed to put the side of his head—where his wound was closed over and healing—directly into the dirt, where the elements of the Earth could penetrate his skull. It turned out that he had actually felt incredibly drawn to lie down in the dirt. You see, soil contains valuable minerals, such as iron, copper, aluminum, and magnesium, just to name a few. In fact, the volcanic soil that grapes flourish in contains the element silica, which is said to have healing properties. I also felt that, apart from being exposed to these healing elements, the Earth would "communicate" to Arnold in some manner and direct him in his life.

When an animal is sick, it will often find healing through the consumption of a particular bush or plant that is available nearby. The plant causes the animal to vomit, clearing the poisons out of its body. Animals also seem to find relief by lying down in the dirt, gaining mysterious benefits from the soil. We should never underestimate the healing powers of nature.

Although it took many months for Arnold to recover, he credits nature as being the ultimate healer.

Paul's Case

Paul called me on the telephone—like Arnold, he was also suffering from a brain tumor. I immediately sensed that there was an issue that was preying on his mind, so I asked him about it. "Oh," he said, "I lost my business a number of years ago, but I've resolved it. I've let it go."

"You may not be physically working in the business, but my impression is that you still have the business working inside your head," I suggested. "It still appears to be a mental strain."

I also knew that there were certain elements that would be useful for him to implement on a physical level. Since the body gets its nutrition from food, I urged Paul not to take dairy products, sugar, or caffeine—all big "no-no's" for serious illnesses—for the next six weeks.

Addictive processes are so strong in some people that they can be a major challenge to let go of, even in the face of serious illness. "But I only drink two cups of coffee in the morning," Paul said to me.

"How is your body going to recover from this illness if you continue to consume toxic substances?" I asked him. "For a short period of time, please leave these items out of your diet. Your body is trying to regroup, and you need to give it a chance to do so."

I also suggested that he drink several cups of a particular South American medicinal tea each day, which would help clean the toxins out of his liver. The liver is the "vacuum cleaner of the body" and does a great job of sweeping and clearing poisons and impurities out of the system. When a person has cancer (or any other illness), an essential part of physical body support is liver cleansing—even healthy people can benefit from purifying this important organ.

When I saw Paul several months later, he still looked toxic. While he'd been disciplined about his caffeine and sugar intake, he hadn't begun to drink the medicinal tea. He looked like a walking time bomb, with poisons circulating within him. I strongly encouraged him to start drinking the tea, educating him about its benefits. I also urged him to seek help dealing with the loss of his business. Even though it had happened many years ago, he had never resolved this issue properly, and it was festering in his brain.

Paul certainly had the capacity to heal, but each of the elements needed to be in place to do so. Once he started doing everything he could to assist his body in the healing process—physically *and* emotionally—he did, in fact, recover.

For some people, being diagnosed with a serious illness can be a death knell—for others, it can be the beginning of a significant spiritual awakening. Serious illness can be a complicated labyrinth of diagnoses, treatments, and circumstances that no single person can decipher. The future lies in the early detection of disease by subtle, intuitive, or technical means. The search continues.

The next chapter will describe the complex and multifaceted nature of the intuitive process.

Chapter 13

Extremely Challenging Cases

Since it's known or believed that I have a healing gift, many people travel great distances to seek my help. Sometimes, though, these people are in really bad shape—I often wonder how people get so far down the road to ill health in the first place. In any case, unrealistic expectations can be placed upon me to perform some sort of "miracle." Here are some cases that have really challenged my intuitive instincts.

Allan's Case

Allan came to me with severe problems—his eyes were so light-sensitive that he had to wear sunglasses indoors. When Allan was outdoors he had to wear *four sets of sunglasses,* one on top of the other. He simply couldn't bear to be exposed to any amount of light. His problem, however, actually related very little to his eyes. Good vision has a lot to do with the liver—that is, a detoxified liver—not one laboring to rid the bloodstream of toxins and poisons, which is what Allan's liver was doing.

According to Chinese medicine, the liver is the seat of anger. Physical body symptoms and emotional correlations have a strong basis in Chinese medicine. Due to their understanding of the body's energy, the Chinese developed a way of linking organs and systems together based on acupuncture meridians or energy pathways. (Traditional Chinese medicine and other alternative disciplines are described in *Alternative Medicine: The Definitive Guide*, presented by Burton Goldberg [Future Medicine Publishing,1998].)

On a spiritual level, eyes relate to *insight,* regarding the higher vision or purpose for one's life—the true destiny for the soul's Earth life. Allan worked behind the scenes in the music industry, assisting musicians in developing their talent. It was clear that Allan had a beautiful heart and was a phenomenal human being who was capable of great things. I suspected that he had many creative gifts of his own that had yet to be discovered, let alone expressed. Perhaps he was so sensitive to his personal vision because it might require personal change or even great sacrifice?

I took a deep breath, tuned in, and began to assist Allan with dietary changes. I started by suggesting that we take the pressure off his liver by eliminating caffeine and candy bars, to which he was addicted. I also proposed supplemental support that was particularly targeted to the liver and the eyes. I had no idea if this would make a difference to someone with such a severe condition, but I always give my best to each person, say a small prayer, and let God do the rest. Two months later, Allan wrote me a letter, updating me on his progress. Here's some of what he told me:

"My light sensitivity is almost eliminated. How do you explain the joy of lying in the sun for an hour without a towel draped over your head? Imagine, I'm able to get my entire face tanned— even my eyelids!—for the first time in 25 years. I had a reunion with the sun, and it truly was a mystical experience."

I suspect that Allan's reunion with the *light* and the *sun/son* will illuminate his true vision for himself and who he is—a child of the universe, or a son of God.

Marla's Case

Marla wasn't brought to me because of any physical problems—she simply would not thrive. It was scary just to look at her, for I didn't see the will to live in this ten-year-old girl. I've rarely seen anyone as nonresponsive as Marla was. Her parents had tried many different therapies to bring her back to a state of robust health—to no avail.

I asked some questions about the different supplements and treatments she was currently taking, and inquired a little about her nutrition, but I knew the answer wouldn't be found in that area. So, I stayed quiet and let my instinct guide me to this statement: "This little girl stays sick to get attention."

Suddenly, Marla's mother started to cry—which people often do when the truth they're carrying around inside is finally identified. "Marla's brother is very precocious and gets all the attention," her mother admitted. *Hmm,* I thought.

Then I was led to the next concept. I said, "She seems to have very little contact with her father."

Marla burst into tears. "My daddy never hugs me," she sobbed. *A-ha! We got it!*

My intuition then led me to investigate electrical influences in Marla's environment. My suspicions were confirmed when I was told that there was a large electric motor, which controlled the air-conditioning in the home, on the other side of her bedroom wall. This electromagnetic stress, I believed, was robbing Marla's body of vital energy, causing her to feel drained or "weird" when she entered her bedroom.

My suggestion was that Marla change the location of her bedroom to get away from the electromagnetic influence. There were three other rooms in the house to choose from—an office, a sewing room, and a guest room—and I felt that Marla should be able to pick the room she felt most comfortable in. Marla picked out her new room, her things were duly moved, and her mother purchased a new set of cotton sheets. In addition, I instinctively felt that Marla should paint the wall at the head of her bed so it looked like a princess bed in a castle. By doing so, Marla would be involved in an exciting creative project, and her will to live would be engaged. Marla loved this enterprise, and truly made the room her own by placing a picture of a guardian angel beside her bed. She said that she always talked to her angel, and it gave her comfort.

These emotional factors, along with the excellent traditional and alternative treatments that she was already following (including nutritional support and a correct diet), assisted her in regaining her health and returning to school. Daily hugs and contact with her father also helped Marla immeasurably, as did the family's decreased emphasis on her little brother, who had all the confidence in the world. Although Marla's case was complex, her will to live was ignited, and she is now a healthy, happy little girl.

Bruce's Case

Bruce sent his photograph to me for a consultation. When I look at a person's picture, a flood of information comes to me—and what I saw was not a pretty sight. First of all, I saw a man who was very overweight, bearing a pale, unhealthy look, and leaning on a cane. Then, since the picture was taken in Bruce's kitchen, I noticed that the counters were laden with all sorts of "no-no" foods. And finally, I could feel a strange, oppressive energy emanating from the picture. Taking all of this into account, I was reluctant to work with Bruce. His situation seemed as if it might be too complicated for me to handle; however, he had just completed a battery of thorough medical tests—which I feel are extremely important before one starts on any course of alternative therapy. All of these rather expensive tests had come up negative with respect to his complaints. Over the past few months, Bruce had mysteriously lost his voice and could hardly speak above a whisper. His joints were also puffy and inflamed—particularly his wrists, fingers, and knees. I decided to give Bruce my best shot over a 14-day period. At the end of two weeks, if there was no improvement, I would know that I'd done all I could, and he would no longer be my responsibility.

In a difficult case like this one, I begin with the basics. The first place I like to start is with the fuel— the food that the person is eating—and the environment in which they live. If I can get some intuitive indications there, I know I'm on the right track. Most people figure that health is an extraordinarily esoteric quest, but in my experience, the biggest clues are found in the simplest areas.

Looking at Bruce's photograph, I immediately

knew that he had several food allergies. Offending foods can trigger immune system reactions, which then contribute to joint stiffness and fluid retention. I hadn't a clue if I could help with his hoarse voice, but we had to start somewhere.

I suggested that for seven days, Bruce eat either broiled chicken or fish, steamed green vegetables, and a little steamed squash at every meal—breakfast, lunch, and dinner. It was a tall order, since I didn't think this guy had ever seen a squash let alone eaten one, but it was worth a try. This kind of program, called "The Caveman Diet," is very effective in reducing immune-system triggers. The principle behind this simple, pared-down plan is to stay away from common foods, and instead eat what is normally never consumed; in this way, immune reactions are inhibited.

At the end of seven days, Bruce reported that his voice was starting to come back, and his swelling was going down. *Eureka,* I thought. *We're getting somewhere.* The body knows.

I then suggested that he continue the plan, without change, for seven more days. At that point, when Bruce called me, I could hear that his voice was stronger. He was delighted to report that his joint swelling had completely disappeared, his balance was more stable, and he was feeling more like himself. As an added bonus, his mind felt sharp and clear, and he'd lost 15 pounds—all fluid! I encouraged him to expand his food horizons, with the addition of more protein choices and some low-gluten rice, for the next 30 days.

Bruce had many pressures on his system, not the least of which was preparing strange and unusual meals for himself. (Fortunately, his plight caught the attention of a chef in a local Asian restaurant, who was willing to prepare just the meals he required.) I could see that Bruce was engulfed by the stresses of an overwhelming and expanding business and was disconnected from his physical body, as many men are. He expected his body to perform just the way it always had—he never figured that it had needs of its own and was going to get his attention . . . no matter what. In addition, his wife had undergone two major surgeries several months before I saw him. I believe this had placed an added burden on Bruce's immune system, which became reactive to many elements in his environment.

On an emotional level, the throat or voice can often be related to lack of expression. I suggested that Bruce convey, in a way that felt appropriate to him, all of the frustrations that he experienced in his business and personal life. If he could find the time, he should also quietly sit every day and listen to what the Divine was calling him to express in his life. In illness, *there are no accidents.* Every part of our physical body represents an emotional issue that needs to be addressed.

To his credit, Bruce followed each one of my suggestions, and to date is enjoying excellent health. When I last spoke with him, his voice was so deep and resonant that I barely recognized him.

I see people in wheelchairs, inching along the sidewalk in walkers, or struggling to get out of a car due to severe pain, and I *know* that they don't have to be this way. God makes things simple, and if we need something, it's never very far away. Yet there are many times when I see people, and even I, as a medical intuitive, can do nothing to help them. This can be heartrending, especially if I know these individuals well.

Craig's Case

Craig came into my life in 1988. When I first heard him speak many years ago, there was magnetic quality in his voice, which made a deep impression on me. He'd been instrumental in encouraging me with my angel doll project, and he was a deeply spiritual person, committed to helping people in all walks of life.

One night, I had a dream about Craig that has frequently come to mind since that time. I dreamed that he was about to undergo major surgery and was covered from head to toe in white bandages. On his shoulder, woven into the bandages, was a small teddy bear. This gave me two clues: I was shown Craig's great need for nurturing, and was also guided to offer lightness and playfulness to the very grave situation at hand. During this dream, I remember speaking to Craig and urging him not to have the surgery. I intuited this dream to mean that he was about to undergo some kind of major spiritual transition— a passage from one place to another, which is why he was covered in white, like an offering.

During this time, Craig underwent difficult challenges—both in his relationships and in his business—which manifested themselves into an illness. My inner knowing was that there was nothing wrong with him, and I urged him to look at his body as a powerful machine that knew what to do to get well. Although his body was taxed, I knew that Craig frequently gave in to his addictions and love of food, alcohol, and entertaining. He had many food sensitivities and environmental allergies. Craig was certainly very spiritual, but there appeared to be much more that he could do to help himself on the physical level.

Unfortunately, in 1998, the dream that I had ten years previously became a reality. Craig had high hopes that open-heart surgery would correct his physical symptoms, but alas, it only addressed part of the equation. To this day, although he's recovering, I believe that the vitality Craig seeks will only be found when he taps in to his body's wisdom and institutes some simple lifestyle choices.

There are cases that are so complicated that nothing short of a miracle can rectify the situation.

Sarah's Case

Sarah was brought to me in a wheelchair. It distressed me greatly to see this poor drooling child with long, stringy hair; curled and limp hands; and a spacey look and sagging head. Sarah had cerebral palsy, and the sight of her brought up a graphic picture of my own daughter, who, due to a difficult birth many years previously, had narrowly escaped the same fate. Yet despite the close call, my children have been extremely healthy, and I gave thanks for them as I looked at Sarah.

This was a difficult case—Sarah was one of The Tricky People—there was little I could do except offer some basic suggestions. She'd taken plenty of antibiotics, and I smelled that distinctive, sweet, yeasty odor around her, so I knew that candida yeast had to be part of the problem. Dairy and sugar were also culprits, and upon questioning her parents about her diet, I found out that it was loaded with macaroni and cheese, bagels, doughnuts, cinnamon rolls, and lots of candies and soda pop. How in the world could I help *anyone* with a diet like that, let alone a defenseless girl in a wheelchair?

I suggested that Sarah's parents immediately start her on a four-week allergy-elimination diet and a candida yeast-eradication program. After four weeks, Sarah's mother's reported to me that Sarah was responding well to the program. Her eyes had cleared, she appeared to be more alert, the drooling had decreased, and she was less fatigued and sleeping soundly.

Sarah still has a long way to go. Who knows if she'll ever lead a normal life? But at least the life that she *is* living can be a little more tolerable. I'm glad I was able to have been of assistance. I also commend her parents for the dedication and love that they showed their daughter. Through Sarah's parents, I observed such love and concern, yet they had completely accepted a very difficult situation—the true meaning of *surrender*. This was truly an inspiring example for me to witness.

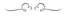

The people described in these cases have all been important teachers for me. I've learned to be grateful for the body that I've been given and for the fact that my own health challenges have been minor in comparison to theirs.

Now, as we move on to Part IV, we'll shift our perspective to the deeper emotional levels of the healing journey.

PART IV

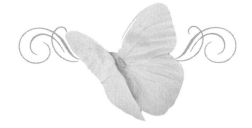

Tuning In to the Emotions and Spirit

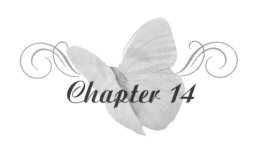

Chapter 14

Emotions and the Immune System

It's now well known that emotions influence the immune system. Cancer, lupus, arthritis, MS, AIDS, and Alzheimer's disease are all serious illnesses affected by a weakened immune system.

Dr. Candace Pert wrote a fascinating book called *Molecules of Emotion* (Scribner, 1997), in which she uses powerful scientific research to document the link between emotions and the immune system. This is probably one of my favorite books of all time, as it speaks of a woman's courage in bringing her medical knowledge, research, and insight into the world against great odds.

A strong emotional body is necessary for a strong immune system. According to Dr. Pert, not only are there *organs* related to the immune system—such as the thymus, spleen, lymph, and adrenal glands—but *every cell* in the body has a component of the immunity blueprint encoded within it.

From my medical intuitive perspective, I've found that when a particular decision is made in life, it must be embodied fully—and accepted by the person on all levels—or physical symptoms will likely manifest due to the misalignment of head and heart. For example, if a person decides to stay in an unhappy relationship or dissatisfying job, or to adopt a certain lifestyle choice or sexual preference, then no matter what their head is saying, their heart and every cell in their body "know" that they must be in agreement or they will be living a lie.

Emotions and decisions that are operating at cross-purposes within can play a huge role in illness and chronic symptoms. As such, it's important that you do all that you can to examine the depth of emotion that you carry, and use it as a tool to strengthen you. Anger, resentment, and unresolved issues can trigger physical reactions—both subtle and dramatic. Seek ways to release these buried emotions— anger directed outward is often a reflection of unresolved issues within. Traditional counseling isn't necessarily your only option. In fact, I often find that people spend unnecessary time in never-ending therapy when there are many effective emotional-releasing techniques available. *Depression*—which we can all feel from time to time—is the opposite of *ex*pression. What is it that you can't express in your life? Find out what it is, grab on to it, and channel this creative expression on a daily basis.

Emotions can ravage the delicate balance of the physical body. I've never worked with anyone who didn't have some emotional component involved in their own health puzzle. Even children can (and do) carry emotional issues from their parents. It's hard to believe, but an unborn child is aware of every emotion and every thought that its mother and father are feeling, expressing, or suppressing. When you carry a baby, remember that *you're guiding your child from the moment of conceptual awareness,* and every thought and action is transmitted to your baby. Even if the circumstances in your life are less than perfect, do your best to be positive about them.

The following cases illustrate the powerful hold that negative and/or buried emotions have on the physical body.

Beatrice's Case

This case tells much about painful memory storage and its link to ill health.

Beatrice had lived for a time in a beautiful, though very polluted, city in South America. She and her husband were involved in a development project, and despite the city's pollution, they enjoyed the cosmopolitan lifestyle. After several years of living in this environment, Beatrice developed a nagging cough that wouldn't go away. No amount of medication or air purification in the home seemed to help. The cough continued even after the couple returned to North America. Then Beatrice's husband died, and she was devastated. Her respiratory condition deteriorated to the point that she had to be hospitalized on a number of occasions. The usual coughing and rounds of medication continued. Like many illnesses, this was of a psychosomatic nature— deeply imprinted in the fabric of the mind.

A few years later, Beatrice suffered a massive stroke. Miraculously, although she was weakened, she recovered quite well. Curiously, during this catalytic stroke, her ever-present cough disappeared completely. It seems that the part of the cerebral cortex that stored the cough reflex no longer held the memory associated with it.

Pat's Case

Pat came to me with continual bleeding in her uterus. The doctors were baffled as to how to help her—a hysterectomy seemed to be the only solution. I stayed quiet, and the voice within me said, "Ask her about her children." It turned out that she was estranged from all four of them. But interestingly enough, Pat was engaged in a relationship with a struggling writer much younger than herself. She was a capable, professional woman who was taking care of this young man—another child. Hence, her life force (blood) was seeping out into the relationship with this man, who was drawing on her strength—and finances—to fulfill his dreams. The lack of communication with her children compounded her problem.

Appropriate supplementation, the addition of red meat to her diet, and specific hormone balancing assisted Pat's physical recovery. On an emotional level, she worked diligently to establish healthy personal boundaries and took serious stock of where valuable energy "currency" was draining out of her body. Over time, she has reconnected with her family and has placed more importance on what matters to her.

Many women who have become separated from their children can experience grave endocrine difficulties. My own mother, for example, suffered from this problem. When she was 46 years old, my father took a position in India, advising doctors and nurses on methods of birth control. In the blink of an eye, our whole family was separated.

My older brother stayed on the West Coast to attend a

university, I was sent to boarding school in Switzerland, my younger sister attended boarding school in India, and my younger brother accompanied my parents. My mother never recovered from the loss of her family unit. Although her husband's job meant that she lived in interesting and exotic places, it was no compensation. She began to bleed to such a degree that only a surgical procedure could correct the problem on the physical level—but it couldn't be fixed emotionally. She'd given her life force to her husband while disregarding her own needs. Several years later, my mother returned to North America to try to gather her family around her and resume a normal life. My father continued his work, this time in Africa. Our family never lived together again.

John and Darlene's Case

Husbands and wives who come to me as clients are very revealing. One such couple stands out in my mind. When I first met John, I received no information about him—he was so blocked that he appeared black to me. In a quandary, I suggested that we work with his wife, Darlene. Ah-ha! Pandora's box opened up—a mine of information was revealed about the woman before me. Darlene's central nervous system was on "red alert," trying to do too much. She was giving, doing, pleasing, and controlling, as well as devoting her energy and power to her husband—he was the black hole into which she expended her energy.

It turned out that John had a serious health condition and needed constant monitoring and around-the-clock medication. Darlene played the responsible role, and because the couple had no children, she'd substituted her husband for a child. She seemed to be completely in charge of her husband's well-being.

Although John's condition was serious, he appeared to be quite calm about the situation, willing to leave the details of his care to his wife, who was on the ragged edge holding it all together. Their relationship appeared to be remarkably unbalanced, and their male and female roles were almost reversed. Something made me ask them about their sex life. My instincts were confirmed in that there was almost a complete lack of intimacy between them. Darlene felt angry and unfulfilled concerning her difficult circumstances, and in the process had repressed her feminine, receptive nature. But more important, she couldn't make love to a "child."

I developed a strategy to calm Darlene's nervous system with protein, B vitamins, calcium, and other nutritional elements. She established a routine to nourish *herself*, and shifted more of the practical responsibilities to her husband.

Chad's Case

Subconscious patterns don't just belong to adults. Eleven-month-old Chad couldn't breathe. His mother fed him cows' milk, which many children are allergic to—especially those with breathing problems. This child was also living in a house with two cats, the dander of which can aggravate sensitive mucous membranes.

On the physical level, dairy products, sugars, and fruit juices were eliminated for two weeks as an experiment to clear the system and Chad's sleeping environment was cleared of feathers, dust, and cats. A specific remedy prescribed by a homeopath was suggested, because if a homeopathic remedy is accurately chosen, it can effectively clear symptoms, due to its ability to effect change on all levels of the body—spiritual, emotional, and physical.

Within three days, Chad's breathing was free and clear. With the physical correction in place, I could see that an emotional problem still remained. On an emotional level, lungs can represent grief. It turned out that Chad's mother had left his father three months prior to our consultation, and the father had no interest in Chad. I believe that this little boy subconsciously felt responsible for this loss. Chad was bearing his own grief, his mother's grief, and the separation from the father that he never really had—all at 11 months of age.

I concluded that Chad may continue to have respiratory problems until his mother comes through her difficult transition and regains happiness and fulfillment in her personal life.

Harmonious Frequencies

Illness results when cells, organs, and systems are out of alignment, or the body's frequency is low. The study of these frequencies, which can be seen with subtle sensing devices or medical intuition, is the basis of energy medicine.

Everything that exists in nature has a resonating frequency around it and within it. All objects, animate and inanimate, are made up of molecules, which are moving particles. The molecules of your body are vibrating or moving at a certain frequency, and the cells and organs in the body of a healthy person vibrate at a higher rate than those of a person who is ill. Thoughts affect the frequency of the cells in your body—thoughts of joy and excitement will cause cells to vibrate at a higher rate. High-resonating frequencies mean that cells are less likely to be affected by disease. Your body is affected by everything that it comes in contact with.

The body knows, and it will show you what makes it feel good and not so good. This principle of the resonating frequency of all living things was the foundation for my clinical allergy-testing work.

If you're looking for the highest levels of health, you need to look for ways to keep your frequency and cell vibration high. Your personal level of happiness is the cornerstone of raising your frequency, thus obtaining optimum health. Once you've discerned the appropriate foods, supplementation, and environmental factors for yourself, they will resonate with your body and assist you in maintaining a high level of energy, health, and vibrating frequency in the body and its organs and systems. Picking the right foods and environmental factors may seem simple and obvious, yet these elements will form the foundation of high cellular frequency. Even the ingestion of a common, supposedly "healthy" food may have a negative resonance for your body. Consequently, when this low frequency is registered by the body, it can feel weak or tired, impacting its high frequency level.

This principle also applies to the people with whom you spend your time. These are people who drain your energy with their negative behavior, words, or attitudes. In time, you'll learn that your resonating frequency is too valuable to let those kinds of people affect it, and you'll choose not to spend time with them.

Music, dancing, and joy will excite cells and raise body frequency, as will any kind of creativity. Being loved by, or in love with, someone, or feeling love in your heart toward all of life, will generate these high vibratory levels. Involving yourself in work or pursuits that you're passionate about will increase frequency. Sometimes being involved in some "necessary" or mundane task will cause your frequency or energy to lower, but taking time out to swim, ride a bicycle, or paint a picture will quickly raise the frequency again. At a high frequency, people appear to stay healthy and more youthful.

I personally carry a small frequency-generating machine that tunes up the frequency of my body when I travel. It can be very useful when I feel drained, tired, low in energy, or if I feel jet lag or the onset of a cold or flu. By keeping my frequency high and tuned up, I function at optimum levels without fatigue.

Deep sleep, meditation, prayer, and our daily link to God will attune us to this high frequency. Positive beliefs also contribute to resonating frequencies. Our thoughts create our reality and also our cellular material. But regardless of our level of spiritual evolution, we still need to be aware of the frequencies inherent in all of the elements of our health program.

The Myth of Spiritual Protection

Just because a person is "spiritual" or religious, it doesn't mean that this evolutionary state will protect them from disease. If anything, spiritually oriented people need to be more conscious of their physical health due to the nature of their increased sensitivity. Such people characteristically become more touchy regarding noise, people—especially negative people—crowds, shopping malls (due to fluorescent lighting and electromagnetic stress), television, violence of any kind, pollution, chemicals, and many common foods and beverages. These perceptive people are being shown, in a very direct way, the effect of their environment, and these revelations assist them in becoming more intuitive toward their bodies' responses to these effects.

These very sensitive and beautiful people are constantly undergoing specific evolutionary changes where the Holy Spirit (or the light of spirit, or the love of God) is increasing and becoming anchored in their bodies. At the same time, their hearts and minds are becoming purified and cleansed. This is called *quickening,* and it requires the development of a pure, compassionate heart—the quest of the spiritual person.

As these changes unfold, these spiritual people are able to transmit and radiate special qualities of love, light, healing, and energy. In fact, their very presence can change a room. Even from a distance, their energy and loving thoughts carry a vast healing capacity. These people do their best to be conscious of their thoughts and actions, knowing the effect that they can have.

Spiritual people are usually very disciplined in mind, but the same discipline must be applied to the physical body and its care. In my medical-intuitive work, I'm constantly amazed at the lack of respect and awareness that so-called spiritual people have for their own bodies—they routinely seem to forget that the physical vehicle is what houses the soul. In so many cases, the health of their corporeal bodies doesn't match the evolution of their souls. Their bodies are very often tired, laboring, and lacking in the vitality that their spiritual orientation suggests. But, because they're so spiritual, or even deeply religious, these people believe that God will protect them from illness. It's not enough to balance the body with affirmation and prayer or to take flower essences and healing oils. It requires that *every* aspect of physical well-being—from correct nutrition and food to supplementation—be taken into account.

I also frequently see spiritual people who constantly process emotional issues and are filled with guilt or self-reproach because they feel that they haven't yet completed their "inner work." Often, the problem isn't even their states of mind—their bodies may be toxic or out of balance on a chemical, nutritional, or hormonal level, thus affecting brain chemistry and emotional perceptions.

The following cases illustrate what I call "the myth of spiritual protection."

Colin's Case

Colin, a man in his 70s, was a well-known healer and teacher, and I was honored to visit his home. He spent many hours each day in meditation, and during the course of this contemplative time, he'd receive divinely inspired information that he wrote down in large books. Over time, Colin had collected quite a library of this beautifully written material. However, he had so completely disregarded his physical body that I was shocked at his condition. Little wonder he was so out of balance, since there were large bowls of candy placed at strategic locations all over his home, and a substantial pot of coffee was continually brewing in the kitchen. His central nervous system was stressed, and his consequent overstimulation meant that his irritation frequently erupted at friends and family members. The vibration that emanated from his body was like a fragmented lightening bolt due to the stress of these stimulants.

The simple solution lay in a change of diet—including a vast reduction in sugars and stimulants—which meant that his physical body suddenly matched his spiritual body. Almost overnight, his formerly scattered radiance returned to healing calmness.

Mandy's Case

Mandy was a spiritual person who meditated a great deal. She suffered from ulcerative colitis, a condition that causes the intestinal tract to become inflamed and covered with bleeding sores or ulcers. This is very often an emotionally based problem, although certain foods can aggravate the situation.

In a clinical setting, we saw many cases of ulcerative colitis. Eliminating sugars, dairy products, caffeine, and particularly glutinous grains—until the intestinal tract recovers—often alleviates the problem. Within a month of following such a food-avoidance program, Mandy's condition cleared up. During this time, she became extremely intuitive and disciplined about the foods she ate, which kept her condition under control. She was also under the care of a competent medical doctor.

Several months later, Mandy had a complete lifestyle change, which led to a huge emotional upheaval. Her two sons left home for college, and her husband left her for another woman. Mandy was devastated. Her home was sold, and until her divorce was settled, her finances were strained. So she went to live with a girlfriend and took a job in a bakery that sold specialty coffees. She became proficient at serving customers and making lattes—as well as consuming liberal amounts of caffeine and wheat-based bakery products, which was her old temptation. Within several weeks on this regime, Mandy had a raging attack of ulcerative colitis and ultimately had to have a colostomy (a surgical procedure to remove part of the large intestine). Mandy mistakenly thought that she'd never be sick again, that God would protect her—even though she disrespected the needs of her body.

Rebecca's Case

Rebecca was a spiritual teacher, adept at assisting others in learning meditation and ways to root out deep emotional blockages. Over the years, Rebecca had become very attuned to her own body, and she took great care to see that she exercised, drank plenty of water, and ate foods that supported her physically. However, she always seemed to be in deep emotional pain, often blaming her family, her past, or herself for the joy that eluded her. It didn't make sense to me that this amount of physical, emotional, and spiritual dedication didn't translate into a greater sense of well-being.

My instinct was that Rebecca's hormones were out of balance. I suggested that she contact a medical doctor skilled in this area. Within a month, she reported that the old "black cloud" of self-blame and depression that had been hanging over her head had disappeared. Miraculously, with this endocrine shift, her life seemed happier and more joyful.

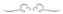

One of the most significant factors in this spiritual and emotional transformational journey—from the human to the Divine—is *fear* and the toll it takes on the physical body. As a spiritual person develops trust in the unknown and in the Divine presence inherent in all of life, the management of fear is an ongoing process. Until this surrender and acceptance process becomes natural and ingrained within us, these fears can wreak havoc on the body, compromising the immune system and leaving it prey to illnesses, allergies, and environmental factors.

In order to be deeply healed, we must forgive ourselves and deal with our emotional difficulties. Chapter 15 gives us tools, when life changes our plans and moves us in the opposite direction, to ride out the crest of the catalytic wave.

Chapter 15

Catalysts and Forgiveness

As a result of illnesses and the breakdown of the immune system—the life force within—people often reflect on the catalytic nature of their disease and how it mobilized them to reexamine what was important in their lives.

A catalyst is a nudge, push, or "cosmic two-by-four" that comes along at an opportune (or inopportune) time to push us in the direction that life wants us to go. Never underestimate its role in your own drama, for a great catalyst can turn a life upside down. It can come cloaked in the guise of an illness; or a financial, family, or relationship upheaval. But no matter what form it takes, you'll be sent on quite an excursion, spiraling downward into the depths of emotion and despair, and ultimately ending up in a place of reevaluation.

Most people wouldn't regard a catalytic event as a grand adventure—they see it as hell. In this process, the universe is trying to get your attention, and it's very uncomfortable at first. But the benefits of such an experience are that you're practically drop-kicked into spirituality, and you'll subsequently develop a compassionate and open heart.

At first, the catalyst is like a quiet nudge—perhaps you'll feel that maybe it's time to make that career move, take that romantic plunge, quit smoking or drinking, or start exercising. The nudge is subtle and quiet at first, and then it becomes louder and louder. If you're a smoker, for instance, you might feel an irritating little tickle in your throat that will graduate to a severe, hacking cough.

Frequently, the nudge stops being subtle and becomes very direct: You wake up in the morning and your wife's not there, a child dies, a car accident leaves you paralyzed, or you're diagnosed with lung cancer or emphysema. No one seeks out these catalysts, but if the message of the wake-up call is heeded, it will push you off your post and move you in a different, usually much more positive, direction.

Bonnie's Case

When Bonnie came to me for a consultation, I took one look at her and knew I couldn't help her. On the physical level, her symptoms had manifested themselves in gross obesity and severe joint pain, to the point that she could hardly walk. I looked at her and knew that it didn't matter what we did in terms of diet or nutrition because these practical measures wouldn't alleviate Bonnie's pain. She was stuck in time due to a catalytic event—ten years earlier she'd been fired from her position as director of a large company. Skilled though she was, the powers-that-be deemed her talents unnecessary.

Bonnie left the company full of anger and resentment. The loss in her life was traumatic, and she sat at home and festered. In the years that followed, she developed a myriad of health problems. Because the little child within her felt so victimized and rejected, she developed a pattern of overeating and negative behaviors to cope, and she was at a loss to figure a way out of her plight.

When we met, I scanned Bonnie's body and suggested that she not see the catalytic event as strictly personal. Instead, I proposed that she try to see the experience as one that was intended to move her forward in life. She'd missed the opportunity that the universe had provided for her to progress, to see that her skills and talents might be needed elsewhere, to seek new vistas and new horizons, and to become aware of a higher purpose. Instead, she chose to stay stuck in a moment that happened ten years ago.

Bonnie's solution was to forgive the person who had fired her, and to let go of the anger and resentment that was keeping her body trapped and immobilized. She needed to see that the entire experience was a setup by her soul for her own growth and learning. She also had to move away from the victimized little child who sought comfort in food. Perhaps then she could do her best to see that she was still young, and she could try to find a place where she could make a difference in the world.

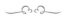

Because all of life and each lesson we learn relates to our spiritual development, the purpose of a catalytic event is to be motivated and inspired to see the difficulty as ultimately useful. In my own life, for instance, the end of a serious relationship provided the catalyst to create relaxation and therapeutic audiotapes, which have comforted thousands of people coping with loss, grief, and uncertainty. It took my own bereavement to understand what was needed to console a damaged human heart. Similarly, my brush with a serious illness provided the background and impetus for my medical-intuitive work. There's no greater catalyst than ill health.

Breaking Apart and Coming Back Together

Several years ago, I had the great fortune to hear a talk given by the late Henri Nouwen, a Roman Catholic priest, and author of *The Return of the Prodigal Son* (Image/Double-day, 1992), as well as many other inspirational books. During this talk, Rev. Nouwen compared the ritual of the communion bread, which is shared by many religious disciplines, to the human condition. His parallel aptly describes the catalyst.

- *Chosen*: The communion bread is chosen, in the same way that the human being is chosen by God to live on the Earth at this time.

- *Blessed:* Next, the bread is blessed as part of the communion ritual—just as the human being, by their very presence, is blessed by God.

- *Broken:* Then the communion bread is broken, as the human being is broken or torn apart in life, through disease, loss, and pain.

- *Given:* Finally, the bread is given to the people in the same way that we're able to reach out and give to people more fully as a result of our losses and sense of being "broken."

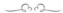

Following are three examples of people who have been "given" to the world as the result of their shattered dreams and catalytic events.

Nathan's Case

Nathan was an interior designer who had a thriving business with many employees. He enjoyed a very impressive lifestyle; for instance, he'd acquired a house, a boat, a summer cottage, and several vehicles. Even though he was surrounded by all of this luxury, Nathan was actually fearful, edgy, and self-absorbed.

Suddenly there was a downturn in the economy, and Nathan's design company was forced into bankruptcy. He lost everything and went into a personal decline that was so severe he needed to be hospitalized. After months of therapy, medication, and deep introspection, he reemerged. He decided to call on all of his former contacts and research alternative employment possibilities in the industry that he'd once enjoyed.

It turned out that Nathan had the perfect set of skills required to execute mediation contracts within the industry, and this turned out to be both very profitable and fulfilling to him. After his long and painful catalytic experience, he now enjoys a calmer lifestyle and a deep appreciation for simple things—including his family, nature, and all of life.

Because Nathan was blessed with perseverance and strength at a core level, he was able to use a key turning point in his life to bring forth the gifts that he had and present them to the world.

Stuart's Case

Stuart came to me in a wheelchair. He had a powerful effect on me the minute I met him. It wasn't so much that he was in a wheelchair that moved me; it was how pure, clear, and emotionally unfettered he had become as a result of his experience.

Looking closer, I could see that, remarkably, Stuart carried no resentment toward his former life or the accident that had rendered him paralyzed from the waist down. Through tremendous emotional and spiritual work on himself, he came to understand that his misfortune could ultimately be used for a higher purpose. He chose to volunteer his time at a local rehabilitation center where he coached people with spinal cord injuries to "get back into life."

Meeting Stuart made any of my own struggles seem insignificant by comparison. This man was sent my way that day to show me the depth of commitment that one human being can make in overcoming a tragedy that would break another person.

Mary Anne's Case

Another example came to me in the form of a beautiful and radiant woman named Mary Anne. Although she had some physical imbalances and weight problems, her smile and very presence could light up a room. She was magnetic. I was fortunate to sit next to her at a dinner party, during which she related how she had survived a very powerful catalytic experience.

One night, Mary Anne had a vivid dream that her two sons would be killed in a plane crash. (Her elder son owned a private plane and was an experienced pilot.) The next day, she discussed the dream with her family and begged them not to fly. Her pilot son said she was crazy—"There goes Mom again with those silly dreams"—and told her not to fear.

A few hours later, as she looked on, the plane

carrying her boys crashed shortly after takeoff and burst into flames. The grief this woman experienced in her devastation was indescribable. It took several years before her life resembled anything close to normal, but she transformed her heartache in a powerful way to help others: Mary Anne volunteers her time at a seniors' center where she spreads her love and radiance to the people who need her.

When I scanned her body, I could see that Mary Anne carried no bitterness or resentment, and her emotional pain had been effectively transformed. The only things holding her back from losing weight were some physical changes, such as limiting carbohydrates and balancing hormones.

As Mary Anne described these horrifying events to those at the dinner table, everyone was stunned. How could any of us survive such a tragedy? Here's what she said: "My faith, my strong belief in God, and the absolute knowing that my children are *safe* gets me through this. I have learned to live my life in appreciation—one day at a time."

How to Handle a Catalytic Experience

If you're living through a catalytic experience, remember that your body is taxed almost beyond its physical limits. Your immune system, which protects the body from viruses, diseases, and environmental factors, is under severe pressure due to the emotional strain. The physical vehicle must not crumble under the stress—you must keep yourself strong as these painful events are unfolding. This experience is the catalyst that draws you deeply into your spiritual nature, and which will ultimately call you to your higher work.

Do all that you can to maintain your physical health in the following ways.

1. **Remember that every molecule of food and drink that you consume is translated into body tissue.** Eat consciously by avoiding any foods and beverages to which you might be sensitive, allergic, or reactive.

2. **Don't collapse into addictions,** that is, over-consumption of sugars, caffeine, and alcohol. These substances will further tax the system and contribute to more emotional hills and valleys. Avoiding these stimulants will give you the mental clarity to make appropriate decisions and deal with the situation. If you must use alcohol, use it as a medicine—sparingly.

3. **Seek help from competent spiritual counselors and mentors** who can assist you in looking at the situation from a higher and wiser perspective. Draw on the strength of friends and family members, or your church, for daily support during the severity of the crisis. Cry. Get it all out. Reach down to the deepest parts of your being, and express your grief with supportive assistance.

4. **Do your best to see that this catalytic experience may afford you an opportunity.** It may be too early due to raw and painful emotions to see it, but in time, the opportunity will be revealed.

5. **Ask these questions: "What is life trying to teach or show me?" "Is life trying to move me**

in another direction?" "Are my skills and abilities needed in another place or location?" Honestly think about the answers that you receive to these questions, as they will be very enlightening.

6. **Look for natural, calming remedies and supplements** to restore and rebuild the body. Some people may require mood-elevating medication or antidepressants during this time. Don't deny yourself this need during such a transitional period.

7. **This too shall pass.** Even the pain of the worst experiences will lessen over time. When you're able to, help others. The gift of assisting others less fortunate than yourself will aid you in looking at your problems from a broader perspective.

8. **Keep gratitude on your lips.** Even when things are at their worst, keep focusing on gratitude. "Thank you, God, for my eyes; thank you, God, for my home; thank you, God, for my friends," and so on, should be continually repeated. The impression that these phrases can have on the mind translates into a soothing, calming effect on the body. When your thoughts turn to fear or deep sadness, reach in and pull out the feelings of gratitude from within. Be vigilant with your thoughts, and keep them as supportive as possible.

9. **Learn to meditate.** Spend time every day being quiet. Close your eyes, and drop into a state of peaceful receptivity where you can

listen to the wisdom of the body and the voice of God within you. (Refer to page 181 to get you started.)

10. **Play relaxation therapy or guided imagery audiotapes** at night as you're going to sleep. These will help calm you down and reprogram your thoughts in a more positive, supportive direction. Also look for the symbols in dreams to guide you. (See page 185 for more on dreams.)

11. **Look after yourself and treat yourself** to massage, soothing baths, a comfy rocking chair, relaxing music, or a cuddly animal. There should be no limit to pampering at this time.

12. **Exercise helps to balance brain chemistry.** As soon as you're able, exercise daily in a manner that's appropriate and healing. Quiet walks in nature or vigorous exercise can assist in finding the inner voice of intuition.

Forgiveness

Once you've experienced a catalytic event, you may find yourself feeling mired in feelings of anger, bitterness, or resentment. One of the best things that you can do for yourself during this time is learn how to forgive. Forgiveness will help you achieve a peaceful state, and allow you to discover the art of surrender, or feeling one with the Divine. It's in this state that our hearts become open and we reach a place of feeling universal love toward all life. When we've been deeply wounded, hurt, or challenged in some way, taking these hurts into our meditations and offering them up to the Divine (asking God for healing and understanding), miraculously transforms these hurts, and ourselves in the process.

In this deep state of peace and acceptance, we're more able to forgive the wrongdoings of ourselves and other people due to the love we feel in our hearts. The art of forgiveness is central to the spiritual journey. As we practice this technique, we're healed on an emotional *and* physical level. The benefits of the forgiveness process are infinite.

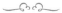

A few years ago, I attended a workshop given by Ron Roth, Ph.D., the author of the book *Prayer and the Five Stages of Healing* (Hay House, 1999). Ron is a spiritual teacher and healer, as well as a former Roman Catholic priest. During the course of the afternoon, Ron led workshop participants in a forgiveness meditation. The sweetness of his words pervaded the room.

"Forgiveness," he said, "means to *give forth*. Give forth what—what do we want to give forth?" He continued, "We want to give forth blessings so that we can feel the same blessings in return."

This was a new and profound concept for me—somehow I was hearing this for the first time. When we forgive and bless a person or a situation with our thoughts, then *we* are forgiven and blessed in turn. It's like a circle—we forgive, and good returns to us.

When we can reach this deep state of forgiveness at a core level, our bodies begin to heal and we're filled with new energy. The simple concept of forgiveness is so tied in to physical body health. When we can't accept a situation or forgive an aspect of our past, these memories stay locked within us at a cellular level. And the same mental program keeps running the unvarying script over and over again so that our bodies continually reflect the mental food that it's being fed. If we could reach for the higher octave and allow life to flow through us, rather than trying to trap life within us, we would experience vibrant health.

An appropriate phrase, which was given to me by a chiropractor friend and mentor, sums up this dilemma: *And you set it up that way.* This speaks volumes about the nature of our not-so-innocent involvement in all of life's experiences. When things are rough, we need to remember that a part of us set things up this way—we chose the conditions on a spiritual and soul level for our growth and learning. I realize that this thought is a conceptual stretch, but it turns the responsibility for the events, choices, and even people in our lives right back to the center—*to us.* When we fully embrace this important concept, there's no blame. The truth is that everything in our lives is a mirror or a reflection of what's going on within.

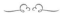

I love the book *The Heart's Wisdom: A Practical Guide to Growing Through Love,* by Joyce Vissell, R.N., and Barry Vissell, M.D. (Conari Press, 1999; **www.sharedheart.org**), which describes one couple's journey relating to the mirror process, which has the specific purpose of reflecting places back to us where emotional work is needed. To paraphrase the Greek playwright Sophocles: "Do not seek to be mastering everything in your life, for the things you have mastered have not followed you." This means that the problems we continue to experience are the issues that we're currently in the process of mastering. When this mastery work is complete, we're free to leave the Earth plane, which is the testing ground for the soul, and evolve to a higher level. The practice of meditation can greatly assist us in the process of personal mastery; it's a simple, yet indescribably profound way to accept any situation in life, *just as it is,* and to feel more peaceful about it.

In order to align with our inner nature and true purpose, we need to establish our spiritual connection—our link to God. When we're peaceful and receptive, inner guidance— or the small, still voice within—can communicate and give us answers to any of life's questions. The answers really do reside inside of us if we just look in our hearts.

The Benefits of Meditation

Meditation should be a cornerstone of any health program. Being able to achieve a deep state of peace on a daily (or twice-daily) basis is better than any vacation. I remember before I learned to meditate that I looked forward to our annual family vacation in a warm and sunny locale. During this time, I didn't have to cook, clean, answer the telephone, or drive a car. I always returned home rejuvenated, but within a few days of my return, I was back to my old stressed-out self again. Then I learned the practice of meditation. I will be forever grateful to June D'Estelle, Ph.D., who taught me this skill. Dr. D'Estelle is the author of *The Illuminated Mind: A Step-by-Step Guide to Spiritual Discovery* (Alohem Press, 1987), and a wonderful meditation teacher.

Thanks to meditation, my medical intuitive ability developed and flourished, and for the first time in my life, I was able to get out of my head, settle down, and feel a deep sense of peace, which was consistently available to me whenever I wanted it. I never needed to go *away* on a vacation again.

How to Meditate

Here's a simple technique that can assist you in becoming peaceful. Find a place in your home—a corner in your bedroom, for instance—that feels peaceful or tranquil to you and where you'll be undisturbed for about 15 minutes.

Some people find soothing background music or the sound of a small tabletop fountain helpful. Sit in a comfortable chair with your back straight and your feet flat on the floor. Assume the yoga position if you like, but it doesn't matter. You just want to be in a position where you can drop into meditation at any time, even if it's just for a few minutes— for instance, while you wait for an airplane, a bus, or an appointment. Eventually, you'll be able to drop down into a meditative state with your eyes wide open.

Close your eyes, and take a few deep breaths to center yourself. Realize that you're special, a beloved child of God. Know that you're one with the Creator, and from that source, all things are possible. Spend a few minutes repeating all of the things for which you're grateful. Send blessings to your friends and family members, and especially to people who are ill and in special need of prayers.

Breathe in and out, in your own rhythm. Repeat: "Centered in the state of . . ." Choose any word that seems right for you, and complete the phrase in a way that feels peaceful and calming. For example, your personal comforting phrase might be: "Centered in the state of peace." But only *you* know the words that will lull you and settle you down.

If the whole phrase seems long to you, try repeating the word *deep* on the "in-breath," and *peace* on the "out-breath." Try this exercise a couple of times, only for a few minutes at first. If your mind wanders and begins to "think," gently take yourself back to your particular soothing words. As you breathe and repeat your phrase, you'll develop a rhythm that naturally takes you into a peaceful state. Soon you'll be able to drop down into this peaceful state and have a mini-vacation whenever you want it. Many of my creative ideas come to me in this serene state, when I've cleared my mind of chatter. Believe me, if *I* can meditate, anyone can.

—⚬⚬—

While you're meditating, there's a technique you can use called "conversing with the illness." This can be useful in determining the emotional reasons for your pain, illness, or weight gain. (A similar concept is explained in *Healing Yourself: A Step-by-Step Program for Better Health Through Imagery,* by Martin Rossman, M.D. [Awareness Press, 1999].)

Take a few minutes to try this exercise. After you've spent a few minutes in meditation and have reached a peaceful state, focus your attention on the area of pain in your body—a sore hip, for example. As you're meditating, ask to be shown what this pain looks like. It might appear as a color, such as an angry red, dark brown, or inky black; or the pain might emerge as a visual image, such as a knotted rope or a dagger. Sit quietly for a few minutes, and allow the image surrounding this pain to come to you. If nothing comes, don't be concerned—some people don't "see" things in their meditations, but they may receive impressions on a feeling level.

After you've established your image—let's say it *is* a knife, dagger, or rope—start to converse with it. Have a chat. Ask the image why it's present in your life at this time. Perhaps there's something that you're doing physically—such as sitting or bending incorrectly, or strenuous exercise—which could be inducing this pain in your hip. Let the painful area communicate with you and tell you anything it wants you to hear. You may receive some surprising insights on an emotional level—perhaps there are some emotional issues related to the pain that you need to address.

Keep communicating with this part of your body until you feel that your session is complete. Then in your imagination, send love and healing to this part of your body—you might even want to imagine a soothing color surrounding it. Tell your body that you're listening to it as it communicates with you. This is a powerful and revealing way to develop your intuition. Do your best to honor and implement the insights that you've received.

Using Affirmations to Heal

Probably the most well-known person to popularize the concept of emotional correlations and physical illness is Louise L. Hay. Her book *You Can Heal Your Life* (Hay House, 1984) has been translated into many languages, and the positive affirmations described within can help you overcome your emotional "stuck places" so that the healing process will be speeded up on the physical level. *All* levels—body, mind, soul, and emotion—must be treated in order to achieve healing. The mind is so powerful that when it hears the repetition of a positive phrase just a few times, it then becomes fact, and the positive behavior is played out in real life.

I've spent many years creating affirmative audiotapes, which offer a useful accompaniment to my medical-intuitive work. The tapes help adults and children get to sleep and feel more positive about life. Imagine having a soothing voice motivating you in a calm and positive way at bedtime. After all, the sleep state is when we restore and rebuild—falling asleep with love and gratitude in your heart will speed your healing process and help you rise above the issues in your daily life. Try repeating these affirmative phrases: "Thank you, God, for my eyes; thank you, God, for my hands; thank you, God, for my job; thank you, God, for my children; thank you, God, for my spiritual growth and all the lessons I'm learning," and so on. The repetition of these phrases of gratitude will help you drift off to sleep quickly and remind your inner self that there's always another way to look at things.

Another wonderful way to fall asleep, especially when life is unbearable, challenging, or seemingly at a standstill, is to say the affirmation: "Something good is always coming," over and over again. And indeed, something good *is* always coming. It could be a friend calling to see how you are, it could be a little bird landing on the windowsill, or it could be finding a lucky penny on the street. No matter how small, the good things are always on the way. Being grateful will keep them coming—always.

The Power of Dreams

Follow your instincts, and allow yourself to listen to your inner wisdom on all levels. After years of working with people with food allergies, I'm convinced that a clear, detoxified body sees, feels, and thinks more clearly. Many people, after they've removed allergens from their bodies, can and do have vivid dreams that can be very revealing as far as health is concerned.

A woman came up to me after a seminar and shared how she'd had a dream revealing polyps in her colon. Tests confirmed that she was right. Her polyps were removed, and thanks to dietary changes, she remains healthy.

Another woman reported to me that she'd been shown a large basket of bread in her dream. It became clear to her that she should stop consuming bread—consequently, her Crohn's disease (an inflammation of the intestinal tract) improved.

Saul's Case

A young man named Saul spoke to me after a workshop. His dream saved his life. Every night for two weeks, he heard a voice in his dream that said, "The green bug is going nowhere!" He woke up each morning wondering what this meant, and every night he had the same dream. *The green bug is going nowhere?* What could this mean? For days he looked at bugs, dead and alive, and none of them were green, nor did this dream seem to make any sense whatsoever.

Two weeks passed, and one day after work, a co-worker at the lumber mill Saul worked at asked if he'd like to go get a couple of beers. Saul agreed and waited while his friend went to get his old Volkswagen Beetle from the parking lot. As soon as he saw the car drive up in front of him, Saul realized the significance of the recurring dream. He was staring at a *green bug.* Just then, a sinking feeling came over him, and he *knew* that he was not to get into that "bug." Saul hastily made up an excuse, saying he'd left his jacket in the building and that he'd meet his friend later at the appointed bar. Two miles down the road, his co-worker (and the green bug) took a curve too wide, veered off the road, and plunged down a cliff.

Dreams speak to us in symbols. Most of the symbols, pictures, or messages are garbled and make no obvious sense. Psychotherapists tell us that dreams are the inner workings of the subconscious, releasing the clutter of the mind. But the symbols of dreams can also be instrumental in understanding emotional blockages, assisting with physical healing, or in foretelling the future.

How to Analyze a Dream

You may wake up from a dream where you're being chased or persecuted. This usually represents a part of you that's trying to get your attention, or an aspect of your personality that's "attacking" you. You'll find that as you clear out your buried emotions and cleanse your physical body, you'll rarely have these kinds of dreams anymore.

Immediately upon waking, make a note all of the images

in your dream. Write down your impressions quickly to get a sense of each dream sequence. Never mind if they seem random and undecipherable. Usually the symbols in a dream are aspects of ourselves, and they speak to us in a language we will hear. For instance, a vehicle, car, or boat usually represents the physical body. A bridge or boat can mean the passage from one physical or emotional place to another. A baby can represent the birth of a new project, not necessarily an actual pregnancy. Water in a dream can refer to the subconscious. As you note down each image in the dream, ask yourself what this could mean in your current situation.

There's no right or wrong way to interpret dreams. The questions you want to ask yourself are: "What does this dream mean to me?" and "What is the deeper, subconscious part of me trying to communicate through this dream?" Ask for clarity regarding an issue in your life to come through a dream. Your desire is to be strengthened, not weakened, by the experience.

It may help to find a person skilled in interpreting dreams. I have a "dream buddy"—a friend who assists me in interpreting my dreams, and I return the favor for her. There are also many useful books to help you get started in deciphering the messages of dreams. I recommend *The Mystical, Magical, Marvelous World of Dreams,* by Hilda B. Tanner (Sparrow Hawk Press, 1988).

Twenty-five percent of dreams are said to be precognitive or foretelling of an event to come. For example, a friend of mine was choosing an apartment. She liked the first place that she saw, but it was facing north and she figured that it would be quite dark and gloomy. That night she asked for a dream telling her whether or not she should take the apartment in this much sought-after building. She awoke from her dream having seen a large stop sign, overshadowed by an eagle surrounded by light. She interpreted this to mean that she shouldn't take the apartment—something better would become available. The dream, which tapped into the deeper unconscious part of her that *knew* what was best for her, had revealed its wisdom.

Two weeks later, another apartment became available—in the same building, but with a west-facing orientation. She was glad that she had trusted her instincts and waited. Her new apartment, filled with light, looked out over the trees to an eagle's nest.

A Dream—and an Awakening

In 1995, I awoke from a dream that foretold a life-and-death situation for me. I dreamed that I was attending a function (an event or experience) at a church (source of spiritual wisdom), and I couldn't decide where to park my car (vehicle, physical body). I was told that I could park next to the minister's car (God, higher authority). In my dream, I quickly evaluated that I wasn't worthy to park my car next to such an important person (not ready to go to God or merge with a higher spiritual power) at that time. The second option that I was given was to park my car in the graveyard (physical death). I could see people stepping out of black cars that they'd parked beside the gravestones, and I didn't feel comfortable parking there. My third option was to park next to a grassy ditch, and I decided that that was the best choice. I noted all the details of this ditch, including the dryness of the earth, the parched, rugged grass, and the yellow dandelions that lined it. When I awoke, I had no way of knowing that this dream, sequence by sequence, would predict an automobile accident that would nearly end my life.

Two days after I'd had that compelling dream, I happened to be making a left turn on a busy country road. As

I put my signal on to make the turn, the thought crossed my mind that this was a dangerous place to be stopping. Just then, I looked in the rearview mirror to see a blue truck approaching very quickly, and I knew I was going to be hit. At the moment of impact, I heard a loud, booming voice exclaiming, *"Life is short and very precious!"* I was in complete *surrender*, knowing that this could be my last breath—I gripped the wheel, and the whole scene lit up with searing white light. Cars were flying in different directions, the truck was overturned at the side of the road, and somehow I managed to end up, upright and unhurt, in the same grassy ditch I'd seen in my dream two nights before.

On a spiritual level, this was probably one of the most dramatic and revealing events of my life. In a nanosecond, I saw the meaning and purpose for our lives and how existence works. Where I was taken and what I was shown at the moment of impact was beyond time and space, and I wish everyone could have this experience. No one would ever disrespect their bodies again, nor would they ever say a mean thing or commit an unkind act. In that one brief moment of time, I was able to feel the anguish of what it would be like to die and not have completed my purpose on Earth. No wonder I'm such a zealot now! This anguish of an uncompleted purpose is hell. Hell is not the fiery furnace we're told about in Sunday school; it's what it feels like to be born for a reason and not take full advantage of the opportunities given to us during our Earthly life.

By the same token, heaven isn't way "over there." Heaven, or the other side of the veil, is right here—just one millimeter beyond our nose. If we put out our hands, they're in the veil. We can be pulled into the veil, or heaven, and we can pull the veil through to us through prayer, contemplation, or meditation. I saw no curving staircases, pearly gates, or Saint Peter standing there taking tickets. It wasn't nearly that romantic, I'm afraid.

In that brief second, I was also shown that it's a *privilege* to have a physical body. I could feel many souls pressing in on me, and I could hear them telling me that they would dearly love to be in physical form, to have another chance to complete their mission here on Earth. These felt like senior citizen souls who would give anything to have one more round on the Earthly plane. According to these souls, we're extremely lucky to be alive and should banish depression and despair once and for all.

The next concept I was shown was that everything has weight and importance. Every "good" thought, word, or action is noted and carries weight; as does every thought, word or action that "isn't good." Nothing is without its price tag; that is, no secrets are hidden, and everything is recorded on the etheric plane. Understanding this concept was life-changing for me.

In this 30-second experience, I was also given the insight that we're only here to love and serve. It doesn't matter what kind of clothes we wear, how we look, how impressive our house is, or the type of car we drive. We could be fat or thin, young or old, plain or pretty. What matters is that we're in loving service to humanity.

As the scene before me lit up, I could see that all of life is interlinked. Human beings, nature, and the cosmos appeared to be thousands of brilliant sparks of light—touching and interacting with each other. Everything seemed to be preordained. The whole scheme showed me that there is a Divine plan, and it appears that our little minds had very little to do with it. I could sense *Divine intelligence* pervading the entire scene. At this level, you could see forever.

It was also clear to me that there is no pain in death. The moment that the body loses consciousness, it's free of pain. We remain alive in *energy,* just not in physical form. At this level, it's true that the soul never dies. But we may experience shock because our physical death may have happened suddenly, without time to prepare, so we have no idea how we got to this level. Fortunately, we're surrounded by helpers—angels, radiant beings, and family members—who assist us in making the transition from one world to another.

There are no accidents, and everything happens for a reason. The good, the bad, and the in-between happens for our own growth. The Earthly plane is about learning the lessons of life as quickly and impeccably as possible. We are here by grace, and our time is short. We could literally be taken off the planet at any time—it's simply not our decision. *We all have a purpose.*

I know that speaking for myself, I immediately saw that I needed to commit myself fully to my purpose, and that there was no time to be lost. To this day, I have dedicated my life to assuring people that there are more reasons to get healthy than just the "obvious" ones.

From this dramatic story, you can see the symbolism of my precognitive dream. My out-of-body experience was revealed in each sequence: No, it was not the appropriate time to go to God or to park next to the minister. No, it wasn't right to park my car in the graveyard. The best spot seemed to be the grassy ditch—with my life intact.

Now it's time to turn over the intuitive reins to *you* and help you discover the voice of medical intuition within yourself.

PART V

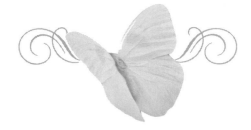

Putting It All Together to Heal Your Family and Yourself

Chapter 16

Honing Your Own Intuition

The gift of intuition regarding the physical body isn't the sole domain of a few select people—it's available to everyone. Any person can hone their skills in this area if they're willing to listen and tune in. After all, we use our intuition to choose clothes, buy cars, seek friends, and pursue hobbies and activities, so why not use it to discern imbalances in our bodies? When we quiet the mind and just listen to the voice of wisdom within us, the task of tuning in to the body becomes easier and easier. Intuition, just like your gut hunches and feelings, will come to you in your own way.

~ ⌒⌒ ~

The following exercises will help you tune in to your own body's wisdom. What you're about to experience will be quite revealing. It can be helpful to do these exercises with a friend. By doing so, you can concentrate on relaxing, and discerning what your body is trying to tell you. All of the answers to life's questions are revealed when the mind is quiet, so don't think or use logic—just relax and let the answers "pop" into your mind from your intuitive level. Keep a pen and paper handy.

Let's get started. Close your eyes, take a few deep breaths, and relax. Ask yourself the following questions:

1. On a scale of 1–10, with 10 being optimum, what is my overall level of health?

2. On a scale of 1–10, how fulfilled am I in my career or chosen profession?

3. On a scale of 1–10, what is my personal level of happiness?

You're now allowing the voice of instinct or intuition to communicate with you. Tune in to answers that are clear, make sense, "feel right," or are "true" for you. If your answers were *below* a 5 for each question, then you probably need to reexamine your life and your choices. If your responses were *above* 5, you're moving in the right direction.

Now let's look a little deeper into these questions.

Close your eyes, relax, and return to question 1. Ask yourself, "How can I increase my level of health to a 10?" Let the answers flow to you from the inside. The inner voice of wisdom will give you answers and ideas to increase your overall level of health, such as changing your diet, drinking more water, increasing your exercise, taking supplements, and so on.

Open your eyes and quietly write down the answers that have been revealed to you. When you've finished, close your eyes and return to question 2. Ask, "How can I increase my fulfillment in my career or outer life?"

Listen to the wisdom of the body as it communicates with you and reveals the truth that you already know. Perhaps it's time to ask for a raise, think about changing careers, take a course, or work fewer hours. Open your eyes and write down the answers you receive, and give thanks to the all-wise, all-knowing part of you that's guiding and directing your life.

Close your eyes again and return to question 3. Ask yourself, "How can I increase and maintain my personal level of happiness?" This is perhaps the most important question of all as far as vibrant health is concerned. What you seek is a very high level of personal happiness. Every cell in your body will reflect the happiness and the joy that you feel within.

Let the answers flow to you as your instinct guides you to clues to your happiness. Should you perhaps buy a boat, swim in the ocean, paint or draw, change careers, review your relationships, let go of an old grievance, or make peace with a friend? Open your eyes and write down your impressions.

This exercise can be very revealing and can be repeated at any time. It only takes a few seconds and will give you a clear indication of where you are and the changes you need to make.

In my own life, when I first did this exercise, my personal level of happiness only came to a 3 out of 10. This certainly wasn't very high, especially since my career offered me plenty of fulfillment. What was making me unhappy was the location of my home. A few months later, I moved to another area of town, across a bridge and by the ocean. When I tried this exercise again, my personal level of happiness had suddenly increased to a 7 out of 10.

Years ago, when I was involved in the fashion industry, I found myself at a crossroads. While I'd initially been attracted to the world of fashion and presentation, over the years it had lost its appeal for me. During a three-day meditation retreat, the instructor led participants in an exercise similar to the one above. As a result of the wisdom and guidance given to me during this revealing process, I took steps to leave the newspaper, and from there I was led to the world of alternative medicine.

—◌◌—

Close your eyes again. Imagine that there's a bird perched above, looking down and observing you. What are you doing? Thinking? Saying? Wearing? Focus and concentrate on the scene. When you have a clear impression of this picture, open your eyes and write down everything that you saw.

Once again, close your eyes, take a few deep breaths, relax, and release that scene from your mind and move to the next one. Remember the bird? This time, the bird is witnessing a gathering of people who know you. They're talking about you and are saying things that are complimentary and useful for you to know.

Observing the scene, the bird asks you how you want to be remembered after you're gone. The group of people that you're watching will give you the answers. As you witness them chatting and talking around you, let the answers from your intuitive perspective come—try not to judge the response; just be an observer. Now open your eyes and write down your impressions.

Take a few moments to thank your inner wisdom and guidance. This is a very important part of you. As you connect more fully to your inner guidance, you begin to trust the responses and refer to the voice within regarding every aspect of your life.

Are you ready for the next step? Take a few deep breaths, relax, and close your eyes again. As you observe the group of people, ask yourself the question, "What steps do I need to take now to see that I'll be remembered for these positive reasons?" Write down the responses you receive.

In my own life, the reason that I was propelled from the world of fashion into complementary medicine had a lot to do with this exercise.

When I was the bird observing myself as a fashion writer, all I could see was a woman in a red jacket (which I frequently wore) running around in a million different directions. When I listened to the group of people talking about me after my death, I could hear them saying that I would be remembered for motivating and helping people. Then, when I asked the question about the necessary steps that I should take to allow these traits within me to come about, it was very clear that I should give my notice, leave the newspaper, and enter a world where I was helping people *and* feeling fulfilled in the process.

The process of trusting your heart or inner guidance takes time and patience. Trust your hunches—just as you currently do with anything in your life. Your intuition regarding your physical body will become just as strong as it is in your career or personal life as you continue to "tune in" on a moment-by-moment basis. The next chapter will show you several methods for tapping in to that inner wisdom.

Chapter 17

Developing Intuitive Accuracy

When I present medical-intuitive training, I usually mention that there are two important pursuits in life. One, I tell the audience, is for the perfect B.M. (bowel movement)—this usually generates a few laughs—and the other, I say, is the quest for the Holy Grail.

The Holy Grail is your spiritual connection, or your link to God. There's nothing more significant than this connection in your life. You can go without food, or even water, for a time, or function without material possessions, but if you're spiritual and wish to live your life from that perspective, you *cannot live* without your inner voice, or the voice of God within you. This is the connection of the heart with the Divine.

As soon as you make this connection, you're never alone. Over time, you'll learn to trust the ways in which the universe is leading you, and during this process, you'll develop all of the gifts you were born to give to the world.

My Holy Grail came to me dramatically in the summer of 1985, when I heard the voice of my angel. I feel blessed to have this guidance every moment of the day. It's always there and a part of me. I could never do my medical-intuitive work without it. If that voice of inner wisdom wasn't available, I wouldn't be able to aid even one person, because I wouldn't be able to "see" or "hear" what to do. I've tried, but I simply cannot do the work without this "hook-up" or guidance from the Creator.

Each day, and with every client, my "internal compass" gently leads me to know how to help: "Ask her about her children"; "Suggest this program, supplement, or practitioner"; "Tell him that he needs to think more about purpose in his life"; "Show her how her buried grief is contributing to her health issues"; and so on. One time, the words "Just suggest that he avoid coffee" came to me, and after I'd shared the suggestion, my client, a man who'd been coping with high blood pressure for years, returned to having normal blood pressure—almost overnight. The depth and level of this guidance never ceases to amaze me.

Inner direction is always very wise and makes sense—giving us that "A-ha!" or "Right on" feeling. I remember a woman coming to me with a problem that wasn't very serious; in fact, it was almost incidental. I stayed silent for a moment to hear about her complaint. Quietly, I heard the words: "Just a simple, common problem." To me, that phrase seemed to accurately and profoundly sum up her rather minor complaint. As I told my client what I'd heard, she laughed, agreed with me, and said she felt more assured.

Wisdom and guidance take time to cultivate and trust. The following pages will give you methods for developing your inner guidance through intuitive accuracy, as your quest for the Holy Grail or your connection to the Divine becomes your most important quest in life.

Simple Methods of Self-Testing

Learning medical-intuitive awareness is incredibly useful, and not just for yourself. You may be called to teach such a method to a friend or family member, and your knowledge of self-testing may save, or substantially improve, someone's life. For instance, last year I had the pleasure of meeting Anna and her two daughters, Cindy and Brin. These two youngsters had a genetic defect that rendered them unable to speak. They had several imbalances that would require "tuning in" to each girl's body for the answers to some tough questions. Both girls were quite mobile but had difficulty reaching out and holding on to objects that were handed to them.

I taught Anna a simple method of self-testing. So far, she's been able to determine all of the foods to which the girls are allergic, and she's learned to tailor their supplementation. In a short time, because of this vital information, her daughters are more alert, have improved digestion, and for the first time, are able to grasp and hold on to objects.

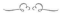

Your desire to develop this awareness will involve the use of some sort of "tool," or method, to tap in to the wisdom of the body. You may have a gut hunch or a "feel" for what might be out of balance, but you'll be able to access deeper levels of understanding if you become proficient in one of the following methods of self-testing.

Muscle Testing

One of the most common methods for tapping in to the body's wisdom is a simple system called *muscle testing,* or *applied kinesiology.* This is a technique that many chiropractors use to discern which muscle, ligament, or joint system might be structurally out of alignment. Thousands of people around the world are using muscle testing on a daily basis; in fact, any good, intuitive chiropractor will use it as part of his or her treatment.

If practiced frequently, muscle testing will put you in touch with your own intuitive instincts. This can be an important first step on the road to becoming a medical intuitive regarding your own body. You should start by locating a local health practitioner who can further introduce you to muscle testing. For practical purposes, in this exercise you'll be learning muscle testing on a *physical* level. If you're fortunate enough to find a muscle-testing practitioner who works on an emotional level, you're in for a pleasant surprise. During this process, the emotional components of physical illness are revealed by the body itself, and translated through the practitioner. Then with simple techniques, they're released.

By following these simple procedures, you can learn to use muscle testing to tune in to your own body. (Keep in mind that the muscle-testing technique I'm outlining here is just one of several that are available.)

1. Take a few moments to calm down and feel relaxed.

2. With your dominant hand, make a circle with your thumb and first finger, as if you're pinching them together.

3. Make a hook with the first finger of your other hand. Place the hook in the center of the circle, and *pull*. For example, make the circle with your right hand and the hook with your left, place the hook into the circle, and give it a slight tug or pull.

In order to discern the inner wisdom of the body, until it just comes to you automatically, you need to ask questions that your body can respond to with a *yes* or *no* answer. Your body will eventually speak to you in phrases, sentences, or discourses—but for right now, *yes* or *no* is what you seek. Your intention is to know what your body really wants. Your intention and desire to *know* will bring the correct answer to you.

Relax and ask the rational mind to step aside so that your intuition is available to respond to your questions. Repeat steps 1 through 3. You're now ready for the next part of the process.

4. Ask to be shown a *yes* or *no* response with your fingers, keeping in mind that the body can only respond with a *yes* or *no* answer. For most people, the hook will slip right through and break the circle for the response *no*, which signifies a weak or "not-good" response to the question. The hook will stop and be contained within the circle for *yes,* or good or strong. So ask the wisdom of the body again: "Show me a *yes.*" What does a *yes* look like? And if your rational mind is out of the way, the hooked finger will stop, or stay firm, in the circle showing you a *yes*, strong, or good response.

5. Then ask the wisdom of the body to show you a *no*: "What does a *no* look like?" And the hooked finger should slip right through the circle, indicating a weak or "not-good" response.

This method is a quick and easy way to get on-the-spot answers to questions regarding items that affect the physical body, such as foods or supplements. Your desire is to know what your body really wants. After you've clearly established your *yes* or *no* indicators, let's put this method into a practical framework.

Putting Muscle Testing to Work

A good way to practice muscle testing is by testing the foods that you eat.

Start by taking about a dozen foods out of your refrigerator or cupboard. Try to choose foods that are single items and aren't mixed together, such as an egg, an orange, a sack of flour, a carrot, a chunk of cheese, or a bowl of sugar.

Next, take your fingers and make your "hook and circle" again. Take a few deep breaths, let your mind go quiet, and establish your *yes* and *no* indicators. Now place your hands over the food item in question, and ask yourself, "Is this substance beneficial for my body?" You want to know the substances that are *beneficial* for your body, not just the ones you *can* eat. After all, you can eat anything—even rat poison—but how favorable is it for your body?

For example, let's say you're testing an apple. With your hook and circle fingers poised over the apple, ask, "Is this substance beneficial for my body?" and await the response. Keep your rational mind out of the way, and test your fingers for the response. Did the hook and circle stay strong over the apple, or did the hook slip right through the circle? Write down your reaction.

Go to the next food—perhaps you've chosen eggs. Note your fingers' response, and then move on to the rest of the foods that you have on the kitchen counter and test them, one by one. Soon, you'll have two categories of food—one beneficial and one not. If you practice the procedure in this way just a few times a day, in only three days you'll have mastered muscle testing for foods.

Now you can learn to "scale" out the beneficial foods and see just how useful they really are for your body. Assume your "hook-and-circle" position again. Regarding the particular food you've chosen to test, ask: "On a scale of 1 to 10, how beneficial is this substance for my body?" The hook will stay strong in the circle until it breaks through at a certain number, as you call out the numbers one-by-one.

For example, on a scale of 1 to 10, this apple is a 1, 2, 3, 4, 5, 6, 7, 8. . . . In this case, the hook stayed strong or firm in the circle until it broke through at number 8. The apple is an "8" on the beneficial-foods scale. Anything that tests above a 5 is favorable to the body—anything below a 5 should probably be left out of your diet.

Use this method to "scale" all of your foods. If there are other items that you don't have on hand in your home, but would like to test them, draw the particular item on a piece of paper or cut a picture of it out of a magazine. You can even think about or imagine those foods and check the level of benefit. In all of my travels and in all of my clinical experience, I've found that there's nothing that can bring a body into balance more dramatically than by eating the foods (the fuel) that the body wants.

Now let's try the same system with your supplements. **Please do not use this method for testing prescription medications. Medications should be adjusted and administered by your medical doctor.**

Most people take far too many supplements, trying to receive benefits from bottles of vitamins instead of from the foods that are right for their bodies. After all, the body processes its nutrition from food, not pills. When I was an allergy-testing technician, there were two test vials that were used every day on every single patient. One was for the tolerance of a certain substance, and the other was for the efficacy of that substance—many items are *tolerated* by the body but aren't necessarily *effective*. On many occasions, sacks of supplements needed to be discontinued, not because they weren't tolerated, but because they weren't effective. Frequently, when people have an ailment, they search for assistance themselves, using information that suggests they take this or that substance for their condition. But because each body is unique, an item that might be beneficial for one person may have no helpful effect for another. Blanket suggestions aren't necessarily the correct solution for every body, which is why you should desire to tune in on an individual basis to find out what your body really wants. The body knows.

Line up all your supplements, assume your "hook and circle" muscle-testing position again, and start asking questions.

1. Hold your circle (dominant hand) and hook (non-dominant hand) over the first supplement bottle and ask the question, "Is this supplement beneficial for my body?" If the response is yes, ask, "On a scale of 1–10, how beneficial is it?" Anything that tests above a 5 is beneficial to the body—anything below a 5 should be left aside for now.

2. Concentrate only on the beneficial supplements at this time, as you'll want to know how many of these you need to take.

3. Ask, "How many capsules/tablets of this supplement should I take each day?" "Is it 1?" Circle breaks. "Is it 2?" Circle breaks. "Is it 3?" Circle stays closed or strong. Then you confirm the body's wisdom by asking, "Is my body telling me that the dose of this supplement is 1 tablet/capsule 3 times a day?" The wisdom of your body, through your fingers, is responding *yes* or giving you a "strong" answer to your question.

   Continue testing each supplement in this manner and record the amounts you're given.

4. Now ask for how long you should take this substance. Remember that the body is only able to respond with a *yes* or *no* answer. For example, ask, "Should I take this supplement for one week?" Yes/no; two weeks?—yes/no; three weeks?—yes/no; and so on, until the "finger circle" breaks. Sometimes the body doesn't know exactly, so supplements should be checked on a weekly, sometimes daily, basis. As you become more intuitive, you'll be able to reach for the bottle and just *know* or feel that it's the right one to take.

There are other ways to use the fingers to self-test, along with the traditional method of applied kinesiology that chiropractors use. You'll find that the hook-and-circle method is very reliable and easy to learn. In about three days, you can expect to become reasonably accurate using this method for testing your foods and supplements.

Using a Pendulum

Another simple way to self-test is through the use of a pendulum. The pendulum has been a common "tuning-in tool" for centuries, and to this day, a dowser (or water-diviner) may be hired to locate water on a property. Mining companies often use dowsers, and oil companies hire dowsers to locate oil stores on maps. The dowser tunes in to the terrain on the map and using their intuitive methods, tries to locate oil in the physical geographical location. Dowsers have an innate ability that assists them in sensing where the water, oil, or minerals are located. They may use a forked stick that quivers or bends over the element being searched for, or they can use the simplest of tools—a pendulum.

Every year, dowsing conferences take place around the

world, and groups of these fascinating intuitives gather together to discuss their latest findings. Anyone can learn to dowse; in fact, I have a couple of engineer clients who dowse or use a pendulum over everything they eat. These are high-powered individuals who build bridges and dams all over the world, and I love the thought of them dangling pendulums over their cornflakes every morning. They're intuitively very adept, and this method of tuning in assists them in knowing what their bodies really want. The use of the pendulum is an important step in acquiring medical intuitive skill, and I teach it at every one of my trainings.

A pendulum is a weighted object that swings back and forth, just like the "tick-tock" mechanism that powers a grandfather clock. A pendulum can be made from a medallion suspended from a chain or a ring looped through a piece of string or ribbon. A common nut, available at any hardware store, also can make a perfect pendulum: Simply hang the nut from a short piece (approximately 16 inches long) of soft string. I have many clients who lovingly "ask the nut" for wisdom and guidance on the physical level.

Make sure that the object you choose for your pendulum is heavy enough to drop down and hang like a weight from the chain or string. If the pendulum weight is too light, it may not swing successfully. Fancy pendulums made from crystal or unique metals are available at health-food stores or metaphysical bookstores. The object of the pendulum is to sense or identify a response to questions regarding the physical body. Your desire is to tap in to the wisdom of your own body and begin to know and understand what it really wants. This is a great way to establish communication with the body—which is trying its best to communicate with *you* on a moment-by-moment basis.

A pendulum, just like muscle testing, can only respond with a *yes* or *no* answer to your question. Your query must be framed so that the pendulum or your sensing device can respond with a simple *yes* or *no*.

Let's get started. In your dominant hand, hold the pendulum so that the weight hangs directly down from your chain or string. There should be approximately six inches of string or chain length between your fingers and the weight at the end. Hold the string with pinched fingers, and in order to keep your arm stable, prop your elbow on a table. Take a few deep breaths to clear your mind and to feel calm and centered. A quiet mind can receive clear, accurate answers.

Now start asking questions. With your elbow propped upon the table, and your pendulum weight dropping directly down from your pinched thumb and forefinger, without moving the pendulum on your own, ask to be shown what a *yes* or *no* indicator looks like. Just as you did in the muscle-testing exercise, your intention is to really know how to tap in to the wisdom of the body.

State the directive, "Show me a *yes*." To what or whom are you speaking? You're requesting that the wisdom of the body or the all-wise, all-knowing part of you respond to your command. Concentrate on the weight/object of your pendulum; your intention is to be shown what a *yes* or *no* indicator looks like to you. For a *yes* answer, the pendulum will probably respond by either moving back and forth or going around in a circle.

Next, concentrate fully on the pendulum, and ask, "Show me a *no*." To be sure that your rational mind is out of the way and you're not influencing the responses of your question, keep a centered, calm focus, and ask again, "Show me a *no*." The pendulum will respond with a different action or movement than your *yes*. It might respond with a counterclockwise circle or a back-and-forth movement. When I demonstrate the use of the pendulum, my *yes* is a circle, and my *no* is back-and-forth. Focus and practice establishing your *yes* or *no* responses so that they become very familiar to you.

Now that you've established your *yes* and *no*, you're ready to ask questions. Let's start with the foods that you most commonly eat. Place all of these foods on the kitchen table, just as you did in the muscle-testing exercise. Once again, use single-item foods. Prop your elbow on the table, and hold your pendulum over each food, one item at a time, and ask the wisdom of your body the question, "Is this substance beneficial for my body?" Observe the response from your pendulum. Does it swing back and forth, or does it make a circle? Some people find that the pendulum may quiver or not move at all in response to a *no*. This response could also indicate a *maybe*. Reframe the question and try again, noting the response to each item of food. Continue to ask the question, "Is this substance beneficial for my body?" for every one of the food items on your table until you *know* which ones are beneficial and which foods aren't.

It takes about three days of using the pendulum in order to become relatively skilled. Most people pick it up very quickly. Some people find the pendulum laborious and slow, and they prefer muscle testing. Your ultimate desire is to achieve body intuitive accuracy without the use of any of these tools, to *know* the answer directly in your own mind. Your desire is to become so instinctive about your body and your world that you're never without answers to your questions; in fact, you want to get to where you know the answer to your question almost before you ask it.

Now let's find out how beneficial all of the supplements you're taking are. Following the same instructions outlined in the section on muscle testing, line up all of your supplement bottles on the kitchen table, and with your pendulum suspended a couple of inches above the supplement bottle in question, ask, "Is this substance beneficial for my body?" Jot down your body's answer, and continue testing all of your supplements in this manner so that you end up with of your beneficial supplements grouped together separately from the not-so-beneficial ones.

As I said, most people take far too many supplements. Many individuals take a great deal of interest in the supplements they're taking without giving much credence to the foods they're eating. The body utilizes subtle and elegant processes to digest and assimilate nutrients from *food*; therefore, if you must take a supplement, try a food-based one instead of one that has been chemically synthesized. The body knows the difference and will usually respond more favorably to food-based supplements.

Just as you practiced in muscle testing, the next step with pendulum testing is to determine, on a scale of 1 to 10, just how beneficial these supplements are. With your pendulum poised above your supplement bottle in question, ask, "On a scale of 1 to 10, how beneficial is this supplement? Is it more than 5?" Yes or no. "Is it a less than 5?" Yes or no. If your body responds *yes* to any of the supplements that scale out more than 5, you can intuitively determine the specific benefit. Just ask, "Is it a 6?"—yes or no response; "Is it a 7?"—yes or no response; and so on.

Now you've determined the specific benefit of each one of your supplements. With approximately three days of practice, you'll be quite skilled at using the pendulum. Always remember to ask questions that your body knows the answer to—those regarding common foods, environmental factors, or supplements, for example. Resist the temptation to ask questions about the future, such as "Am I going to win the lottery?" or "Am I going to marry the man/woman of my dreams?" The body only knows what is appropriate and beneficial *in the present moment,* and the future is just speculation.

Pulse Testing

Another simple method of testing the body for offending foods, beverages, and substances is called pulse testing. When I was first tested for all of my food allergies using provocation/neutralization (P/N) testing—a process where allergens are injected under the skin—I was acutely aware of a raised pulse rate from certain substances. I found out later that a raised pulse can indicate a potential "immune reaction" to a certain allergen, thus contributing to unwanted symptoms.

Begin by taking your thumb and first finger and placing them around your neck so that you can feel the pulse in your carotid arteries, which are the main blood-supply channels to your head. These places on your neck should be easy to find, and they'll have a strong steady beat. Get to know what a normal pulse in these areas feels like. You can also find a pulse in your temple point, located about two inches above your eye and to the right (or left, depending on which eye). Try placing your fingers on the temple, and feel the pulse of the blood flowing under your skin. Get to know what a normal pulse feels like in this area as well. You can also test your pulse in your wrist, although for some people, this may not be as easy to detect.

About 20 minutes after you've eaten or drunk anything, put your fingers on the pulse point that you're testing. If you've consumed something that the body is allergic or sensitive to, your pulse rate will increase, signifying that the body doesn't like what you've just consumed. The offending food has triggered an immune reaction and has signaled a message to the heart to increase the flow of blood through the arteries to dilute the toxins or poisons in the bloodstream.

At this point, noting your elevated pulse rate, just ask yourself, "What have I just eaten, drunk, or come in contact with that could be causing a reaction?" Think back to what you had at your last meal and put your clues together. This helps to develop your own intuition about the foods that are right for *your* body. When you discover the offending substance, leave it out of your diet and challenge yourself, again taking note of your increase in pulse rate. It usually takes between two to four hours, sometimes even longer, for the pulse rate to return to normal.

When you become aware of your food allergies and omit offending items from your diet, your blood pressure will often return to normal levels. Pulse testing is also useful to detect sensitivities to chemicals such as tobacco smoke, perfumes, and cleaning compounds.

Challenge Testing

Another type of easy testing, though somewhat time-consuming, is called a food *challenge*. As I've previously stated, the most common allergies or sensitivities are caffeine, sugar, wheat, dairy (particularly milk), corn, and soy. These should be the main items to focus on in your challenge. Other common food sensitivities include eggs, tuna, citrus fruits and juices, certain fish, shellfish, nuts, and spices—you may want to test these items as well.

Take all of these items out of your diet for five to seven days to give your body a rest and to clear your system. Now, one item at a time, with a day of separation between each item, challenge yourself to the effects of each offending food. First thing in the morning, on an empty stomach, sit down to a very large portion of each food and nothing else—a half cup of sugar one morning, two cups of strong black coffee the next, two pieces of whole wheat toast the following morning, two glasses of milk after that, and so on. Within 20 minutes of consuming your challenge food, if you're allergic or sensitive to it, there will be a reaction. You may notice that your heart pounds, your pulse races, your stomach doubles up in knots, you have intestinal gas, or you develop a headache. Note your reactions, and take this item out of your diet, as it's an offending food. Then carry on normally and eat the rest of your meals that don't contain sensitive items. You've done your research—your body *knows,* and it's showing you how to become more intuitive.

Everyone wants their test answers to be reliable and exact, but this takes time and constant practice. Over the years, my accuracy has developed as a result of working with thousands of people, as well as having an understanding of how certain elements and processes work in concert. When this inner guidance came to me like a bolt of lightning in the early 1980s, my skill and direction were very clear from the outset. However, with practice, my gift has become more finely honed. Being able to drop in and out of a receptive state, receive guidance, and make sense of it forms the basis of the work that I do today.

Your desire is to see and discern the body with new eyes—from an emotional, spiritual, and physical perspective. The body isn't just a moving mass of flesh and bone, it's an elegant and complex set of systems, which, when given the right elements in the right combination, according to its directives, will function optimally for a lifetime.

Other Beneficial Treatments

After you've experienced the benefits of a medical-intuitive assessment and have followed the "basics," you're ready to investigate the refinements—other forms of "fine-tuning." At this point in your healing journey, I would suggest that there are two very important areas that should be strengthened: One is the heart and the other is the liver. All of the simple suggestions that we've been discussing can strengthen these organs, but there are additional ways to enhance the process.

The heart is obviously one of the most sensitive and vital organs in the body. If it stops, *nothing* goes! The heart can be taxed in many ways, due to stress, poor diet, lack of exercise, and genetic predisposition. Emotionally, the heart has the capacity to be broken and healed many times in its life—but not physically. There are many ways to strengthen the heart: Avoiding stimulants, lowering cholesterol, and specific supplementation to assist in removing plaque from arterial walls can all help. When the heart is strengthened, all physical body processes obviously benefit.

The emotional heart is very sensitive and resilient; on this level, it needs nurturing, love, calm pursuits, and the feeling that it's being heard and acknowledged in all decisions.

The liver is considered to be the seat of anger in Chinese medicine. On the physical level, it's a major chemical factory, performing vital functions such as filtering the blood, storing important nutrients and energy-producing sugars, detoxifying the system, and assisting in the digestive and elimination process. As with the heart, cleansing and strengthening the liver can improve overall body function.

On an emotional level, the release of buried anger and resentment is an important next step. At this time, I suggest that you consult with a skilled practitioner who can assist you with deeper levels of detoxification and support.

Acupuncture, homeopathy, bioresonance therapy, massage, and hands-on healing will all work more profoundly when you've completed your "basics" and your body is free of surface toxins. There's a virtual cornucopia of healing methods available to us today. If you can afford it, I suggest that you receive massage or foot reflexology once a week; and continue to have chiropractic adjustments, network chiropractic or eye movement desensitization and reprogramming (EMDR) to release old emotional patterns; acupuncture and biokenisiology treatments; and Reiki or some other form of "hands-on healing" treatment on a regular basis.

If cost is a factor, try trading treatments for something

that you can do, such as baby-sitting, accounting, or carpentry. Couples can take turns giving each other foot or body massages. Everyone should learn muscle testing or kinesiology—then we would rarely need to look for help outside ourselves. Muscle testing is a unique and simple way to determine which foods, substances, and emotions could be affecting the physical body—and it's absolutely free!

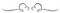

Now that you've had the opportunity to detect items that may be contributing to your own symptoms, in the following chapters, we'll discuss some of the common imbalances that may be affecting the people you love.

Chapter 18

Tuning In to Your Children

I f your child is suffering from mood swings, behavior problems, recurring stuffy noses, ear infections, bed-wetting, or learning difficulties, don't despair—let your intuition go to work.

Although it's alarming that so many children today are displaying aggressive behaviors (disorders such as attention deficit and hyperactivity abound) it's not a mystery. These aren't unusual or "special" children who are from another planet—they're just kids who are out of balance. And thanks to my clinical days and the many miracles that I've witnessed regarding children, I'm heartened to say that there are answers for these problems, and most of them are quite simple.

If your child has been diagnosed with ADD, ADHD, dyslexia, or any other labeled disorder, I recommend that you first read a small but very helpful and important book by Dr. William Crook, M.D.: *Dr. Crook Discusses Alternatives to Ritalin in the Management of ADHD* (Professional Books, 1997). You should then analyze *everything* in your child's environment before you start on a long, expensive, and painful quest for treatment. Start by taking a good look at your child's bedroom. If you're looking for ways to clear your child's breathing passages, the bedroom usually holds important clues in this regard. For instance, check for dust and feathers, and keep pets away. (Refer to the guidelines in Part II regarding creating an environmentally safe sleeping area.)

Keep in mind that these so-called mysterious mind disorders, such as ADD, seem to respond well to a special brain-integration technique called Educational Kinesiology, or Edu-K, now taught in many schools and colleges. A skilled Edu-K practitioner uses muscle testing to determine which parts of the brain aren't integrated or "switched on" for enhanced learning or positive behaviors. Then a series of simple exercises are performed by the child (or adult) and, miraculously, the brain starts to function as it was intended. Contact the Edu-K Foundation at 800-356-2109 (or e-mail: **edukfd@earthlink.net**) for information or a practitioner in your area.

I remember reading a story about dyslexia in a national news magazine. In the article, there was a picture of a ten-year-old girl surrounded by a maze of lights and high-tech equipment. I use this picture in all of my medical-intuitive trainings to show, from visual signs alone, that her "brain disorder" has nothing to do with a label. In my opinion, this girl, who lives and copes with her "disorder" somewhere in North America, could be greatly helped by some of the methods we've been examining in this book.

Your Child's Environment

One of the most well-known pioneers in the area of food and environmentally allergic children is Dr. Doris Rapp, M.D. Through her work, Dr. Rapp has been a great mentor and inspiration to me throughout my many years of involvement in environmental medicine, and her groundbreaking treatments have assisted countless families in living normal lives. Parents everywhere feel enormously grateful to her.

In her book *Is This Your Child? Discovering and Treating Unrecognized Allergies in Children and Adults* (Allergy Relief Foundation, 1-800-787-8780; **www.drrapp.com**), Dr. Rapp documents actual cases of food-sensitive and environmentally reactive children who have returned to normal health by adhering to food-avoidance programs, candida yeast eradication, and specific treatments. Think about anything that your child may be eating, breathing, or coming in contact with that could be causing these adverse effects, and know that many children improve quickly when offending foods, additives, chemicals, inhalants, and molds are removed from their environment. Dramatic improvements also result following the eradication of candida albicans yeast—the proliferation of which is present in almost every child that I see.

Dr. Rapp's book *Is This Your Child's World?* (Allergy Relief Foundation, 1991) addresses the issue of poor quality air, shoddy lighting, and exposures to chemicals and toxic cleaners in homes and particularly in schools. Her video, *Environmentally Sick Schools* (Allergy Relief Foundation), gives us a revealing glimpse at some of the chemicals and other factors that our children are exposed to on a daily basis in their learning environments, and what can be done to help. (The excellent resources by Dr. Rapp are listed in the Suggested Reading section of this book.)

Children with behavior problems are often extremely sensitive to chemicals. Consider changing your laundry soap to an unscented one, and try not to wear perfume around your child. Chlorine, gasoline, and petrochemical fumes can also trigger reactions, so make sure that there's no leak in your natural-gas stove or furnace. Examine the cleaning fluids that you use around your child: Are they strongly scented? Also check for highly fragrant cleaning compounds used to clean your child's school. This takes time, but it's so worth it. The plan is to eliminate substances that could be altering your child's behavior. After you've completed this research, you'll become very intuitive as to what could be triggering reactions.

Clearing Children's Systems

Children today are bombarded with many elements that can be upsetting to their fragile systems. Parse out these elements before you accept a label for your child's problems. Don't cease in your quest for answers, and use your intuition. Parents are often highly perceptive about what's affecting their children, and they're usually willing to implement any changes that might bring about relief.

When I worked in clinical settings, the most common problems that I saw in children were tummy aches, stuffy noses, recurrent ear infections, and behavior and learning problems. Most of these concerns are usually easily corrected on the physical level when food allergies are identified and candida is eradicated. An important question to ask is, "Could my child's symptoms be the result of repeated antibiotic treatment?"

The most dramatic place to start in helping your child is with a short test or clear period. This needs to be a seven- to ten-day span of time when you or someone responsible can monitor everything that's put in your child's mouth and everything your child comes in contact with.

Start with sugar and dairy products. In a clinical setting, I observed that these two allergens seemed to cause the most adverse reactions. Keep a careful focus on the effects of these two substances on your child. Remember that this is an experiment, so during this time, it's wise to keep your child out of stores and away from friends' houses in order to avoid temptation.

- If your child is having behavior or learning problems, a stuffy nose, or recurrent ear infections, eliminate dairy products from their diet for seven to ten days. Dairy products include milk, yogurt, cheese, cottage cheese, and ice cream. Keep in mind that eggs aren't dairy products. Butter, although it is a dairy product, is usually permissible because it contains almost no milk solids. It's the milk solids in dairy that can trigger an immune reaction in the child.

- Believe it or not, the inability to concentrate and irritability are common signs of an allergy to dairy products in children. Bed-wetting can also be a result of this allergy. In addition, you'll find that when you eliminate dairy from your children's diet, they'll have a better attitude, and surprisingly, more energy in the mornings—it won't be as difficult to get them out of bed. The immune reaction to dairy products in some children is multifactorial.

- Behavior problems in children can also stem from a high sugar intake. During your seven- to ten-day test period, eliminate sugar in all forms—even honey and fruit juices, which have high sugar or natural sugar content. Fresh fruit, in moderation, is permissible.

- Read labels and watch food additives, colorings, and dyes, as many children react strongly to these elements. Avoid candy and any other products containing sugar for this same short period of time, of course. All other foods are permissible, except for eggs, peanuts, oranges, corn, wheat, or tuna, which are common sensitivities.

During this clear period, you'll probably notice positive changes around the fourth or fifth day. Even though you're observing favorable alterations, keep going for the full test period. Write down the differences you're seeing and ask your children how they feel. Have them look in the mirror as the puffy eyes and dark or red circles under the eyes start to disappear. Ask them to comment on new and positive behaviors. As an added incentive, draw a "smiley face" or place a colorful sticker on each day of the calendar that has been clear or allergen free. Continue to reward your child and note positive behaviors.

After your child has completed the seven- to ten-day test period, you'll be ready to begin what is known as a *challenge period*. This is when you introduce each of the offending or allergy-provoking foods into your child's diet one item at a time.

On your first challenge day, for example, sit your child down to a large glass of milk. Wait approximately 20 to 30 minutes and watch for reactions. You might witness a child who doubles up in pain from a stomachache, or one who's running around wildly or acting inappropriately. You might notice that your child's nose is running, or they might be wheezing or coughing, or have flushed cheeks or swollen eyes. Be observant—it won't take long before these reactions become apparent. And during this process, you're developing your own medical intuition.

The following day, challenge your child with the next offending substance—perhaps this time it's sugar—and watch for reactions. If your child has severe behavior problems, I suggest that you videotape them in their calm state prior to conducting a challenge. After the offending or allergy-provoking substance has been introduced and you observe the reaction, film the child in their agitated state. The video will serve as a poignant reminder to the child of the consequences of eating off their program. Try using alternative milks such as soy, rice, or almond milk in your child's cereal. Goat's milk may be tolerated; and soy, rice, goat, or sheep cheeses can be useful alternatives. When parents are concerned about calcium intake, I suggest that they research other food-based sources of calcium, such as green leafy vegetables, whole grains, or almonds, as well as supplementation designed for children.

Rice or rye bread, millet or amaranth bread, or alternative flour pancakes can be used in place of wheat bread. Corn or potato chips, or rice cakes, although not particularly nutritious, are useful substitutes for snacks. Children with wheat allergies are especially challenging, because wheat or flour is *everywhere*.

Since milk allergies are so prevalent and fruit juices are so loaded with sugars—natural and otherwise—these beverages should be avoided and reserved for occasions when there are no alternatives. Teach your children to love water and know its value. Water, I tell children, is the most incredible magic drink in the whole world. They look at me with eyes of wonder as I relate its healing properties to them. If we educate our children early to the benefits of water, they'll drink it as a matter of course.

In the long run, after you've observed your child's behavior and symptoms improving, keep exposures to offending foods, toxins, airborne inhalants, and chemicals minimal. Build up your child's immune system with positive reinforcement and appropriate supplementation.

I've personally witnessed positive dramatic changes in countless children. Parents will exclaim that they finally "got their son (or daughter) back" when offending foods and chemicals were eliminated from the environment. If your child has been given a label of any sort relating to hyperactivity, behavioral problems, or learning disabilities, look to these guidelines before you accept a label and a lifetime of challenges. These children can and do turn around when we ask the question, "What does this body want?" Maureen is a prime example.

Maureen's Case

Ten-year-old Maureen was brought to me because she had difficulty learning. She was in a special class for children with such disabilities, and despite all the psychological testing and techniques that her parents tried, she didn't respond. Maureen was bloated and overweight, and according to her mother, seemed to be constantly eating—especially sweets and carbohydrates. "We just can't seem to keep her out of the cupboards," she said.

I, of course, suspected the usual food allergies. Because I'd witnessed so many children just like Maureen in the clinic, I suggested that she implement a candida yeast-eradication program for four weeks, discontinuing sugar in any form, and dairy products for the same period of time.

Within a month, Maureen's mother called to say that her handwriting, spelling, and reading had improved to the point where she was ready to integrate into a regular classroom for certain subjects. Her teachers were stunned by the change in Maureen.

"Our prayers have been answered," her mother said. "She's a different child."

The Emotional Connection

Children become reactive when their immune systems are weak or compromised, and with all of the changes in our society and the restructuring of the family, there are many pressures on children. Fears and insecurities regarding divorce and disruption in the family, as well as violence at school, gather in the subconscious. Therefore, we need to look at the emotional issues behind the reactive child: What's the relationship like between their mother and father? Are there financial pressures on the family? Could sibling rivalry be a factor?

If your child is having behavior problems, take a look at yourself as a parent. Often a disruptive child may be acting out your repressed behaviors. You may be holding it all together on the outside, but on the inside you're feeling overwhelmed, angry, or frustrated in some area of your life. Could your child be acting out some of your unexpressed emotions?

Children model what they're exposed to. At this point in our history, there's no safe place, and in this fast-paced world, many children are the casualties. On a higher level, when we look at the difficulties our children are experiencing, especially in North America, we need to look at the situation symbolically. I believe that the collective "mother" is absent—there's no one looking after the children—consequently, they're running amok.

I also believe that young people today are overstimulated; and that violent television programming, movies, video games, and electronic toys *do* have adverse effects. Children are also becoming more sedentary—and thus more obese—due to countless hours of passive entertainment and lack of physical exercise. Like adults, children need space where they can turn off the world, unwind, spend time in nature, or just curl up with a good book. Do all that you can to implement strategies to rectify these problems.

Sweet Dreams

I believe that we collectively haven't yet tapped in to the power of the sleep state, one of the most opportune times to reprogram the mind and consequently influence the attitude in positive ways. Years ago, my "inner guidance" led me to speak to my own children in a loving, quiet voice as they were drifting off to slumber and after they'd fallen asleep. (My method is outlined in my book *Mommy I Hurt, Mommy I Love You.*) I based this on the age-old method of sleep-learning and the power of affirmations. The results were both immediate and remarkable. Here's a brief description of my technique.

Kneel beside your child's bed as they're going to sleep. After you've discussed their day, read a story, or said prayers together, stroke their back or the side of their face with your hand as you talk to them in a loving manner. Even though you may be tired or frustrated from the events of your own day, stay focused on what you're doing. *You* will benefit from this technique as well.

Repeat positive, loving phrases over and over again in a soothing, repetitive manner until your child falls asleep. It helps to repeat as many "I love you"'s as possible, such as: "Mommy loves you. Daddy loves you. Mommy and Daddy will always love you. You're safe and secure." Repeat this several times. Then list all the people who love your child, such as: "Your sister, Mary, loves you; your little dog, Sammy, loves you; your Grandma Harriet loves you; your piano teacher, Mrs. Jones, loves you; your Uncle Joe loves you; everybody loves you," and so on. Keep naming all of these people, and the fact that they love your child, as much as you can. Say anything positive that comes into your mind, and repeat these loving, affirmative phrases over and over for about 10 to 15 minutes while your child is going to sleep.

This is powerful reprogramming of the mind, for you're reaching the deep subconscious part of your child's brain and are planting seeds for "good" to grow. I call this method the "giant eraser," because it appears to erase the negative thoughts and events of the day. As you follow this procedure, you'll notice that your child will appear more peaceful, and their breathing will be even and calm. Don't stop when they're asleep—keep talking for a few more minutes.

Repeat this procedure night after night for just a few minutes, adding in as many positive thoughts and phrases as you feel guided to say. Watch your child over the next several days. It won't take long before you'll notice subtle, or even dramatic, attitude changes in your child. They'll seem happier, more willing to help, and more agreeable. This positive programming supports children as they're growing up, and prepares them for the challenges that we're going to discuss in the next chapter—becoming teenagers.

Chapter 19

Special Concerns for Teenagers

It can be a challenge to reach today's teens with respect to the effects of food and the environment. Teachers tell me about their frustrations with students who consume excessive amounts of soft drinks and sweets and then detract from valuable class time with inappropriate behavior and inattentiveness.

In my clinical experience, I often saw desperate parents who were seeking any kind of help that might shed light on their child's behavior and learning problems. Under these circumstances, it was often difficult to find a compliant teenager who was willing to stay on track with dietary manipulation or supplementation. There had to be a motivating factor, and vanity often played a vital role in this regard. Teenagers are frequently consumed with their appearance, especially their skin and their weight. When a teen ceases the consumption of sugar and dairy products, their skin will usually improve dramatically, which is often the only impetus necessary to get (and keep) them on any sort of a healthy food plan.

This reminds me of a man I met at one of my lectures. He showed me a picture of his son, Ryan. I saw a boy with a big toothy grin—he looked like a personable fellow, but his face was covered in spots. Fortunately, I'd seen this kind of picture many times in the clinic, so I knew what needed to be done. Ryan's father was surprised to hear that the mere avoidance of sugar in any form, as well as fruit juices and dairy products, for a few short weeks might yield results. This man went home and passed on the information to his son. Ryan's father later reported that his son's skin was clearing nicely and would only erupt if he drank milk or consumed sugars in excess. Once again, the body knew what to do.

Also keep in mind that most teenagers in North America have been exposed to a lot of antibiotics, usually for ear and respiratory infections that they suffered from as little children. Due to exposure to antibiotics, the normal flora in the digestive tract can become imbalanced, and candida yeast may be responsible for a teenager's constant desire for sweets in any form. A candida yeast-eradication program can easily correct this problem.

Teenagers and Weight Issues

In the case of overweight teens, the same principles that apply to adults is also useful to them. Identify food allergies and leave them out of your teenager's diet for a 14- to 30-day period, and have them eat heartily from all remaining foods. In most cases, the weight will drop right off, even without exercise. On rare occasions, hormonal imbalances may be part of a teenager's weight problem; if that's the case, you should take your child to a specialist for careful correction. But weight is mostly related to sensitivities to common foods.

Sheila's Case

A woman came to me for a consultation. After her own assessment, she showed me a picture of her teenage daughter, Sheila, who aspired to be a concert pianist. Since Sheila was a child prodigy, she often had to appear in front of an audience for piano recitals, and she was very self-conscious about her weight. Sheila had tried calorie counting, liquid diets, celebrity diets, fasting, and exercising, to no avail.

I suggested that her mother isolate the offending foods that were making Sheila's immune system react so negatively. Naturally I pointed to dairy products and sugar, and suggested that these items be removed from Sheila's diet for four weeks. I later heard back from Sheila's mother that her daughter had dropped the excess weight effortlessly, was now much more confident about performing in front of an audience, and felt much better about herself.

Rebellion

Body piercing is an interesting phenomenon among young people. It's a "tribal" practice designed to make a statement and to gain the acceptance of the group or clan. While it may be appealing to some, there can be effects from body piercing that are worth noting.

The body is comprised of subtle energy systems and meridians, which is the basis of acupuncture. When the body is pierced on one of these vital energy "lines," it can weaken an entire organ or system. With respect to ear piercing, for example, if the acupuncture point related to the bladder on the earlobe is punctured, it can have the long-term effect of bladder weakness. I suggest that before body piercing takes place, consult with an acupuncturist to determine a desirable and energetically "safe" location.

On an emotional level, when you observe a teenager's life, it can be fraught with many changes and stresses, such as peer and parental pressures, boyfriend/girlfriend issues, low self-confidence, and fear of the future. The immune systems of teenagers—unless they're the happy-go-lucky, hang-loose types—are assuredly under constant attack.

My suggestion for parents is to leave pertinent information around the house, say as little as possible, love your teens a lot, and when they come to you asking for help with dietary issues, conduct a short "let's see what happens" test. Expose them to the same food-clearing and challenge regime I talked about in the last chapter—when your teen's body becomes the laboratory, they'll have a much better idea of what they're doing to themselves. And remember never to discount the power that vanity has in the world of a teenager!

Now let's move on to the particular issues that women of all ages face.

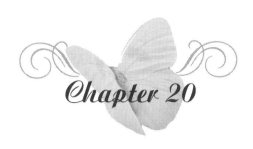

Chapter 20

Women's Issues

Women have some specific needs that can be addressed intuitively. All through our childbearing years and beyond, our bodies experience wonderful (and sometimes not-so-wonderful) changes and challenges. Let's start with a subject that most women face in their lives at one point or another.

Birth Control

Population control was the life work and specialty of my father, who spent many years in developing countries assisting medical teams with methods to curb their mushrooming populations. In our own society, birth control is probably the most frustrating and complex issue that a woman of childbearing age has to face. Since so many women, married or not, are sexually active today, this can be a frequent (if not daily) dilemma.

Birth control pills, like any other medication, aren't for every woman. All too often, I see beautiful young women suffering from the negative effects of the Pill. Obviously, these women have the best intentions, as birth control pills are highly effective in preventing unwanted pregnancies, but because the delicate female hormone balance can be upset by the Pill, there are often unwanted side effects as well.

I look at these pale, tired, and often depressed women and ask myself, "Why is it that we can land a man on the moon, yet we haven't figured out an effective way to prevent unwanted pregnancies?" Even my father, who specialized in regulating populations and was aware of every method of birth control available, had no concrete answers to that question.

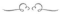

A young woman named Janelle, who was on the Pill, came to see me. She was only 25, but had suffered from low energy, depression, and horrible skin eruptions for the three years that she'd been taking birth control pills. Her skin had become so scarred that she was worried that she might never again experience a clear complexion. She had no idea how her hormone cycle worked, and food allergies and candida yeast compounded her problems. Because of her obvious sensitivity to the Pill, I suggested that with her doctor's help, it might be worth researching other options for birth control. Janelle seemed surprised, as if it hadn't occurred to her that she had a choice in the matter—and many young women are exactly like her in that regard.

As mothers, we must openly discuss with our daughters the subtle changes and messages our bodies give us during all the stages of our monthly cycle. (Men also need to become more educated and supportive in this area.)

Because they'll be dealing with this ebbing-and-flowing for about 35 years, women should become more familiar with their own particular cycles. For instance, did you know that the chemical makeup of our saliva changes at various times of the month? When a woman is ovulating, there are obvious patterns that appear in the saliva and can be seen under a microscope. For some women, education about and detection of these patterns can be a welcome solution to the birth control problem, since just knowing when they're fertile gives them the power to allow or prevent the conception of a child. Kits and instructions for reading saliva are now readily available through some alternative-health magazines, holistic doctors, and health-food stores.

After purchasing such a device and studying her saliva patterns, Janelle, like many other women, is no longer depressed, enjoys clear skin, and has regained power and knowledge regarding her own body and its cycles.

Menopause

This stage of a woman's life is very interesting. Not long ago, the menopause years signaled a certain decline and displacement for a substantial number of women. This isn't so today, when women are encouraged to be just as engaged in life as they were in their youth. I dislike the idea of being considered "over-the-hill," a crone, or a wizened-up old woman. I prefer to focus on the menopausal woman's stature, confidence, wisdom, and grace, and on making the most of her assets—inside and out. Optimal body weight, nutritional absorption, bone density, and physical appearance, as well as a passion for living—are all the achievable goals of healthy menopausal women. This is our time.

When I look at a menopausal woman on an energetic level, there are certain things that I look for. One is an overall vitality and a strong auric or electromagnetic field. Another is an excitement or zest for life, and a link to purpose and passion.

During menopause, which usually begins in a woman's late 40s and continues in its full-blown state until her late 50s, several changes start to happen, including emotional fragility, hot flashes (or "power surges" as they are lovingly termed), night sweats, and weight gain. A menopausal woman can feel as if she's on shifting sands, always changing, and feeling as if she has no solid internal reference point. Trying to balance a menopausal woman from a medical intuitive perspective is like trying to balance a moving target.

The visual image regarding a group of menopausal women is a line of several ladies standing in front of me. I'm writing suggestions on pieces of paper for each woman, who takes the paper and goes to the back of the line—only to be in front of me again 20 minutes later, requiring a whole new program. That's how changeable a menopausal woman is.

During the pre (before), peri (in the middle of), or post (after) menopausal years, there are many changes taking place that we need to be aware of. Let's take a closer look at what the body is going through.

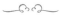

You've probably noticed that during menopause, there tends to be weight gain, especially around the waist. This extra band of fatty tissue, which hangs like an apron around the middle, is called *omentum,* and is a natural part of every-one's body. Men are just as prone to this "middle-aged spread" as women, and it's due to endocrine imbalances. We'd like the omentum to have a little *momentum* and not be so prevalent, so we try to hide this stored fat by wearing oversized shirts or baggy pants. Yet when I look at a menopausal woman from an intuitive perspective, I like to discern her food allergies and sensitivities. By identifying food allergies and avoiding offending foods for a period of time, the omentum level can decrease.

Another part of the excess-flesh equation is the dreaded cellulite. We don't have to be menopausal to accumulate this lumpy material—women (and men) of all ages are plagued with it. I find that most women who know and deal with their food allergies, particularly to dairy and caffeine, have almost no cellulite.

Weight gain in menopausal women can also be related to high estrogen levels—which can be affected by soy consumption. Soy is a very common allergen because of its indigestibility, and it may be linked with endocrine imbalances. So if you're overweight, you might want to decrease your soy intake for a period of time as an experiment. Knowing your food allergies, increasing exercise to burn off excess omentum, and keeping carbohydrate grams low (refer to Part II of this book) can be useful ways of getting your weight under control.

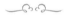

The next thing I like to look at in a menopausal woman is the level of absorption through the digestive tract, particularly the small intestine. All of the foods a person eats (and the supplements they take) are absorbed through hair-like structures called villi, which line the surface of the small intestine, rather like blades of grass or a shag carpet. In some people, particularly CNS types, these villi can be worn down or shorn off due to poor diet, food allergies, and sensitive gut linings on the physical level. And on the emotional level, worn-down villi can be compounded by a lack of confidence; and giving away power and attention to people, places, and things outside of a person. In a menopausal women, a small intestine filled with healthy, robust villi means that her cells, hair, nails, skin, and eyes will be supplied with high-quality nutrients that serve to build up, rather than break down, organs and bones. You don't have to be intuitive to see this breakdown—your quest will be in understanding the role of nutrient absorption, physical energy, and cell tissue repair in a menopausal woman, be it yourself or someone else.

_⟋⟍⟍_

Seeking perfect endocrine balance is another important component of being a healthy menopausal woman. During menopause, the endocrine system—comprised of the pineal, hypothalamus, pituitary, thyroid, parathyroid, and adrenal glands, as well as the reproductive organs—is changing and slowing down. Due to hysterectomies, we may be missing body parts related to the reproductive system, but the endocrine glands are still functioning, albeit not the way they were in our 30s and early 40s. The glands need to be encouraged to function optimally as we continue to age. This can be accomplished with diet, nutritional supplements, and hormone compounds, both natural and synthesized. This is a delicate balance, but with expert help, it can be achieved.

What you're aiming to do is feel good physically *and* emotionally—calm, stable, and balanced, with a great sense of well-being, boundless energy, high libido, and zest for life. It's not impossible, especially considering that there are many medical doctors, practitioners, and experts whose life work and expertise focus on balancing hormones. Don't rest until you find someone who can assist you in this area.

The menopausal woman is constantly changing on an endocrine level. Because your cycles and symptoms are always shifting, you'll be working with your practitioner on a regular basis to achieve balance. It's unlikely that the same hormone substance will help you all the way from the peri-through the post-menopausal years. I've also found *What Your Doctor May Not Tell You about Menopause,* by John Lee, M.D. (Warner, 1999), to be a very useful reference regarding hormone fluctuations at this stage of life.

Some hormone compounds cause side effects—you should know what these side effects are. Don't settle for weight gain and feeling crummy. Keep researching and asking questions. The future for the menopausal woman lies in specifically tailored hormone compounds, which are calibrated on an individual basis to match her changing endocrine system.

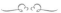

Bone density for menopausal women is also a concern. Look at your family history—did your mother or grandmother have osteoporosis? Do you drink coffee or soft drinks, which can leach minerals out of the body, contributing to bone loss? Use your instincts and isolate your food allergies. Learn to look inside your body and see if the villi in your small intestine are soaking up your nutrition. Take a good-quality, highly absorbable calcium. Get a blood test done, which can reveal proper calcium utilization in the body. Have a urinalysis scheduled to detect any calcium loss through the urine. Exercise daily at a routine that you enjoy, but one that builds bone density as well. Weight-bearing exercise, for instance, has been known to help build bone density.

There's a tendency in the menopausal years for some women to give up on their appearance and let themselves go. But this is a time to look, feel, and be your best. Research your most flattering clothing styles and find out which colors bring out your best features and help you to "come alive." This is for your own well-being. Keep in mind that you're delivering a message every time you present yourself. You're making a statement and attracting people and experiences to you as a result of how you feel inside.

During my time as a fashion writer, I frequently saw women get makeovers. As each woman was transformed from head to toe on the outside—with new clothes, makeup, and hairstyle—the woman changed on the inside. As a result of her new look, she would invariably became more confident, outgoing, and happy about herself. In my seminars for menopausal women, we focus on setting a new stage and demystifying the challenges of the menopausal years.

Menopause isn't a time to shrink back and remain shadowed in obscurity—it's our time to shine. Our Earthly days in human form are numbered. They don't stretch lazily in front of us as they did before we reached the 5-0 milestone. The unique piece of patchwork that we've been called to create here in this world needs to be completed before we move on to a higher level of consciousness. The notion of *destiny* is operant at this time, meaning that we need to respond to our own unique call to make the world a better place. This is why the menopausal years are so exciting and important. They're the forerunner of our later, elderly years when it's essential that we stay healthy, live full lives, function independently in our own homes, and stay out of institutions. In the next chapter we'll discuss this important phase of life.

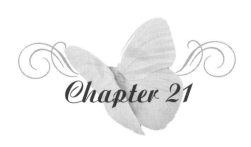

Chapter 21

Health and the Elderly

Elderly people have the capacity to turn their health around at any time, providing their physical bodies and organs have the ability to do so, and they have the personal motivation to make the necessary changes. The following stories underscore this premise.

Yvonne's Case

I consulted with Yvonne, a 72-year-old woman suffering from arthritis, over the telephone. Nevertheless, I could immediately detect candida albicans yeast. Even over the phone I can detect that sweet, sickly smell. I suggested to Yvonne that she avoid all sugars, wheat, and fermented products for 30 days. I received this letter from her sometime later:

> In just a few weeks on your suggested program, even with "cheating" on my plan a few times, the difference in how I feel is amazing. I wake up in the morning not nearly as stiff as I

*used to be. I can now get out of bed without
having to oil my joints before moving. My hips
used to ache no matter what, and now they
feel so much looser and sturdier. I can walk up
and down stairs almost easily, rather than
experiencing my usual struggle. I also find that
although my habit for sweets hasn't been broken completely, my taste for them has changed.
I no longer enjoy the old tastes the way I
remember—for instance, I don't really like ice
cream or candy anymore.*

*Thank you for your insight and help. I hope
to continue to lose weight; get rid of outdated
cravings; and regain energy, health, and joy.*

Claire's Case

Claire came to me seeking help because her
hands were so crippled by arthritis that her fingers
were "clawed," and she couldn't stretch them out
straight. Although she was 80 years old, she was one
feisty lady, and she peered down on me with hawk-
like eyes. It was hard to look beyond this intimidat-
ing presence.

I suggested two remedies for Claire. One was to
eliminate wheat- or flour-based products for a short
period of time, since, due to immune reactions,
wheat allergies can be responsible for joint stiffness.
The other suggestion was to take sugars out of her
diet. It seemed as if all Claire ate was bread and
sugar. It turned out that she hated her mother, and
ate candy constantly in defiance of this woman—
who had long been deceased.

Three days later, Claire returned to the health-
food store where I was doing consultations to show

me her hands. In just 72 hours of staying away from wheat and sugar (but eating heartily from everything else), she could hold her fingers out straight. Such is the wisdom of the body, which knows what to do at any age.

Beth's Case

Twenty years before I met her, Beth lost a child to cancer. Over the years, she'd dedicated her life to spiritual study, and spent several hours each day in meditation and prayer. Yet the devastation from her loss had taken a tremendous toll on her body, and her deep emotional pain had manifested itself in constant sore throats.

The throat is the connection between the head and the heart, and I intuited that Beth was having a conflict between the two. Her head was telling her that she'd worked through the emotional pain of her daughter's death, but her heart knew differently. Beth had never fully expressed her grief through crying, deep release, or talking it out in psychotherapy. Therefore, all the repressed anger she felt toward the world for her grief materialized into endless throat pain. After all, who could recover from such a tragedy?

I suggested some nutritional support to strengthen Beth's immune system, as well as more protein in her diet to increase her stamina. I also recommended an exercise called *toning,* which involves visualizing the area in a person that needs healing, and then humming a specific musical note, one that feels appropriate, into the painful area. The toning of the note is also accompanied by visualizing a healing color surrounding the area in question. This is a helpful and effective way of releasing pain, both on the physical and emotional planes.

I also had a sense that various environmental factors could be irritating Beth's throat. The climate she lived in was very dry, so the addition of a humidifier in her bedroom, and increasing her fluid intake assisted in soothing her throat as well.

I commend elderly people who are willing to dig deep and process emotional issues. Once Beth finally did this—and also combatted her problem on a physical level—her throat stopped troubling her, and Beth found herself finally at peace.

Nutrition can be a tricky subject for elderly people, as they've often lost interest in cooking for themselves. I'm not elderly, yet even I know how they feel. No wonder older folks tend to get into the "tea and toast syndrome." Cooking, necessary as it is, can become very tedious. If you look at a "mature" person's typical diet, it's usually highly starch- or carbohydrate-laden, since breads and carbohydrate snacks are easy to prepare. As you know, carbohydrates break down into sugar in the bloodstream, and these sugars, when not balanced with protein, can make the person feel jittery, shaky, spacey, light-headed, and even forgetful. In addition, many elderly people are plagued with the candida yeast syndrome, which can be a factor in Alzheimer's disease. Therefore, it can be very helpful to limit the use of sugars on a daily basis— a small amount of fresh fruit should be eaten instead.

Older people are often deficient in protein, probably as a result of how time-consuming it is to prepare. If you're caring for an elderly person, make sure that protein in some form is part of each meal, as increasing the consumption of animal protein can help with stamina, blood-sugar regulation, and resulting emotional balance. Good-quality supplementation can also be useful.

Thanks to television advertising for adult diapers and pads, it's now common knowledge that bladder frequency and leakage is a major problem for people of advanced age. Caffeine, as well as citrus juice, can be very irritating to the bladder. Caffeine can also break down the delicate sheath or coating around nerves; leach vital minerals out of precious bones; and add to agitation, irritation, and shakiness. Elderly people, especially CNS types, shouldn't drink coffee, black or iced tea, or any product containing caffeine. Since caffeine is a stimulant, simply avoiding it can make a significant difference to an elderly person's balance, gait, and state of well-being.

I feel blessed to have worked with so many elderly clients, and I can vouch for the fact that the body knows how to obtain health at *any* age, and elderly people aren't too old to discover their food allergies and learn how to work with them.

As I grow in years, I become even more attuned to what will keep me strong and healthy as I live my life of purpose. I look for role models in elderly people—I spend time observing their level of compassion, sense of humor, and forthrightness, along with their love of nature and devotion to their families. I hope that when I reach their stage in life, I will have developed a deeper sense of what's truly important, and will have fully shifted my perspective to the higher octave.

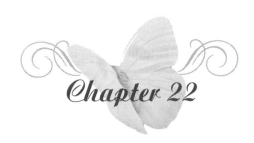

Chapter 22

Reaching the Higher Octave

Given all the "feel-good" reasons for optimum health, none are as compelling as the notion of destiny. In order to anchor a deep respect for the physical body firmly in our minds, and to give us the motivating factor for achieving optimum health, we must look to the idea of purpose and calling as the driving forces behind our intentions. It's time to live life from *the higher octave.*

Sure, it's great to feel healthy and alive, and when we feel this way, we have the energy to do just about anything. But just feeling good is not enough. When destiny gives us a project, however large or small, we need to have a healthy body to carry out our purpose and mission, for the passion of our calling does as much to excite the cells in our bodies as it does to keep our souls fulfilled. As we take the steps to uncover our unique talents, the journey—and the experiences we have along the way—takes us to our ultimate goal of completing our calling in this lifetime. A sense of purpose can be a powerful motivating factor for releasing addictions, maintaining a peaceful heart, letting go of blame, and seeing the bigger picture.

Andrea's Case

Andrea, a beautiful, capable young woman in her mid-40s, came to me for a consultation. She'd spent eight years training for a job she didn't like—consequently, she had low energy, lethargy, and pains in both of her ankles and heels. I had a sense that despite what her mind was telling her, she'd veered away from her true purpose, and the flame of passion was missing from her life. I did my best to assist her from a nutritional and supplemental perspective, and her energy did improve, but her real Achilles' heel—where her pain was actually located—was in direct proportion to her lack of fulfillment in her job. Frequent meditation assisted her in finding her inner voice, and she was led to calligraphy as a way to balance her daily work with a creative outlet while awaiting a new career direction. I also suggested that she read a book called *Pinpoint Your Destiny: Discover Passion, Purpose and Calling By Using Your Natural Talents,* by Curtis Adney. This is a wonderful resource for those of us who need guidance in finding our dreams and making them reality.

Andrea is now much happier and healthier—on *all* levels.

Illness begins when the spiritual part of our lives is disregarded. We stay in jobs we don't like or relationships we've outgrown, and we're content to feel old, lethargic, and in pain. When we realize that we have a finite number of years on this planet, living life consciously and purposefully takes on new meaning. We need to align with the universe, as it has something bigger in mind for us. When the soul prompts us to move forward, we must be ready to take the ultimate leap of faith—and this takes courage.

The healing journey, like life itself, can be unbearable and challenging at times. To stay grateful—even when life is falling apart—to develop trust in the unknown, to be positive when in pain, and to remain calm and in the present when there's nowhere to turn, takes great discipline and mastery. But the rewards for this work are great, for when we release large chunks of anger, resentment, and bitterness, the real gift is that our meditations become deeper, sweeter, and more revealing, and we develop more compassion and understanding in our hearts. As a result, the facets of our individual "diamond personalities" are finely polished— emitting light, radiance, energy, and love that have far-reaching effects.

Learning from Others

I feel blessed to have many inspirational role models who have shown me, through their writings and teachings, how to stand firm and persevere in the face of challenge. I often think about the following figures, who I consider stellar role models, and wonder: *Who were these people that they could be so loving, compassionate, and spiritually aware, despite their own personal circumstances?* What examples they are for the rest of us, who are still so incredibly self-possessed.

For me (and many other people), the Dalai Lama, the spiritual leader of the Tibetan people and Buddhists worldwide, is one such hero. In his book *A Flash of Lightning in the Dark of Night: A Guide to the Bodhisattva's Way of Life* (Shambhala,1994), the Dalai Lama points out that all human suffering is the result of our expectations and subsequent disappointments when we realize that life is beyond our control. He says that focusing on praise in order to avoid criticism, pursuing gain to avoid loss and pleasure to avoid pain, or seeking acceptance rather than experiencing obscurity, keeps us locked in the wheel of struggle. Discipline, spiritual practice, and a compassionate heart are the only ways to liberate us from this cycle. Surely if this man, who, along with his people, has suffered so much adversity, can look at things positively, we, who have undergone so little by comparison, can do the same.

It's hard to be perfect, or even close to it. Like you, I have moments when I'm at my worst. At such times, I draw on the inspiration of Mother Teresa and the way that she was able to look at each and every sick or dying person in front of her with eyes of compassion and the soul of a saint. That's quite a tall order, but surely I can perceive someone or a situation with new eyes if I can reach for the higher octave. The Virgin Mary, the Divine mother, is also an inspiration to me. Often the image and presence of Mother Mary will be there to comfort me when I feel alone or confused. I just imagine her beautiful, soft, steady, loving presence, and her blue robe surrounding me. That image alone can settle me right down.

Jesus can also be a powerful inspiration. When looking for answers and direction, this entity, felt by people worldwide, can be a life-changing example of how to live a better life. A remarkable book that describes the attributes that Jesus possessed has helped me to live from the higher octave. It's called *The Twelve Conditions of a Miracle: The Miracle Worker's Handbook,* by Dr. Michael Abrams (Abundance Media, 2001).

Or take, for example, what happened not long ago to a friend of mine. John was having a particularly stressful time in his life and went into a small church to pray. This place had always felt peaceful and comforting to him, so he knelt at the altar for a while and found himself returning to serenity. On his way out, although the light was dim, he could see two homeless men curled up asleep on the pews. He thought about waking them up and sending them out, but something made him stop and consider what Jesus would have done in this situation. Jesus, he felt, would have let the men sleep, and John walked out of the church knowing that he'd done the right thing.

When we draw on the strength, wisdom, and guidance of these spiritual masters, our own personal level of self-mastery is elevated. Through this process, we find our distinct inner voice. Also keep in mind that you can never know how someone else may be inspired by *you*. For instance, I gave a talk in Los Angeles a few years ago, and I mentioned how strongly optimum health is tied to spiritual purpose. Several weeks after my presentation, I received a letter from a man who'd attended the lecture. He said that he'd given up chain-smoking after grasping this concept. He said knew that he needed a strong physical body in order to complete his purpose as a spiritual songwriter. I had no way of knowing that the words I spoke would make such an impression on someone whom I didn't even know.

Similarly, I'm not just influenced by larger-than-life role models. For instance, it seems that the moment I start to dwell on a certain difficulty, I'll see someone in a wheelchair, or with far greater challenges than I'll ever have to face. This immediately brings me back to the realization that I have so much to be thankful for.

To Everything, There Is a Season

Several years ago, I had the unique opportunity of working in a beautiful heritage church. It was set in a little cove at the edge of the ocean, surrounded by trees and a lovely garden. Inside, there were dark wood beams, lush red carpets, and ornate stained-glass windows. It was a very popular location for weddings—but for all the brides that walked up the aisle, there were just as many coffins that were carried down. Working at a church gave me the opportunity to witness the extremely dramatic and transient nature of life. As I saw these important chapters unfolding before my eyes, I once again realized that life is too short to waste. This experience continually forced me to reset my inner compass and focus on what really matters in life.

Remember that as we take the true journey from within, from the ego to the soul, there are many hills and valleys to traverse. In fact, the day I finished writing this book, I was reminded of this concept. That day, I received word that a friend of mine had died. She wasn't an old person, but for many years she'd disregarded her body's signals, to the point that she lost her life far too early.

I don't profess to know the mysteries of life, but in my opinion, there are three kinds of death. One is the "timely death," where the person passes naturally on to the next realm after living a full life on this plane. Another is what I'd term a "catalytic death," where someone is plucked before their time and placed in the hands of the Creator with no advance warning, leaving those behind to ponder the meaning of such an event. The catalytic death, if it's to have value, is to push or motivate someone who's been impacted by this loss to make a significant contribution to the world. The last kind of death is the "needless death"— the slow, chronic, crippling, cell-by-cell demise of so many people who choose not to heed the wisdom of their bodies. This is what happened to my friend, and, like a tree in the forest, she fell long before her time.

To all of you who wish to see the fruition of your own dreams, please keep yourselves healthy. Call upon your intuition, your inner guidance, and your body's wisdom to keep you on track. Let this instinctive part of you show you the way to all the choices that are right for you—as well as appropriate practitioners who can help you—until each layer of your "health picture" is clearly revealed.

It's my earnest hope that I've laid before you many of the practical steps that you can use to reach the level of health that's rightfully yours, because in my experience, the attainment of health is usually a very practical matter.

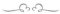

Writing this book has been a tremendous pleasure. I've shown you how to identify your own body systems and potential imbalances, as well as gain insight into the most common, yet powerful, places where ill health can occur. I hope that the discussion of case histories motivated you and shed some welcome light on your own physical symptoms. I urge you to discover the emotional reasons beneath your health picture and work with them so that they become your greatest teachers. And finally, my deepest desire is that this book has taught you to become your own medical intuitive so that you're prepared to help yourself and your family—now and in the future.

Just remember that *the body knows.* In the quiet of dreams, and in the spaces between the busyness and the noise, let your body speak to you. When, like a beacon, your body is healthy and filled with enough energy and vitality to light up a room—and your heart is imbued with the power of love—your intuition and connection to the Divine will inspire you to bring out your best and offer it to the world.

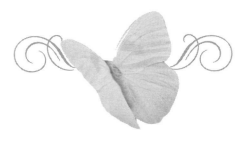

APPENDIX

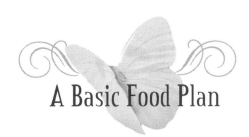

A Basic Food Plan

Following is a basic, easy-to-follow meal plan. (This program is not meant for children.)

- If you're pregnant or lactating, consult your doctor before starting any program.

- Use fresh, organic, whole foods whenever possible.

- Read labels.

- If you're not trying to lose weight, add carbohydrates (starch) to every meal. Personally, I like to keep my carbohydrates low; by doing so, I have consistent energy and mental clarity.

- The idea with a plan such as this one is to keep it simple. You don't have to take things down to the "last gnat's eyebrow" or be hyperdisciplined and inflexible as far as foods are concerned. What you're mainly trying to do is avoid sugar, caffeine, and the common food allergens; give your digestive and immune system a rest;

and feed yourself healthy, satisfying meals. Eat the foods that your body *really* wants.

Drinks

- Drink at least eight glasses of purified or spring water per day.

- Try herbal tea or coffee substitute, with a drop of natural sweetener.

- Don't drink *any* dairy products.

- Consume fruit juice sparingly.

Breakfast

- Cook eggs any way you choose. Try them omelette-style, with steamed and chopped vegetables, such as cauliflower, broccoli, zucchini, green beans, ½ a carrot for color, and so on. Cook and drain the vegetables first, before adding the beaten eggs. Add salt, pepper, spices, and herbs as desired.

- Remember that eggs are an allergen for some people. This sensitivity can manifest as nausea, headaches, digestive problems, rashes, or mood changes. Because eggs are created through a hen's reproductive system, they're a hormone component—I've actually seen people break down and cry when they were injected with egg extract during allergy testing in a clinical setting. However, most people who are allergic to eggs are aware of it.

Some Breakfast Alternatives

- Try organic turkey or chicken sausages—or salmon, poultry, or meat from the previous night's dinner—with or without steamed vegetables. If you're not allergic to soy or beans, try a tofu-and-vegetable scramble.

- If you're on the run, two whole rye crackers (such as Wasa) with almond butter is a good choice.

- Don't eat fruit with breakfast. I occasionally enjoy some fruit during the day or after dinner, but I time it to several hours after a meal.

- Stay away from carbohydrates at breakfast and lunch. I notice that I feel better, and have more energy, mental clarity, and stamina—and no food cravings—if I do this. On weekends, if I'm at home, I enjoy a slice of 100 percent rye toast with my breakfast. Since I have a wheat (flour) sensitivity, I stay away from it whenever possible, as wheat in any form makes me tired, and frequent exposures to it make my joints stiff.

Lunch

- Make a large salad comprised of a variety of interesting lettuces plus chopped green vegetables of any sort. (Some people are sensitive to the cabbage, or mustard food, family. These include broccoli, cauliflower, cabbage, Brussels sprouts, kale, and so on—check the *Food Family* list on page 277. These vegetables can cause digestive problems such as discomfort, gas, or burping.)

- Add any of the following "goodies" into your salad, such as red pepper (watch tomatoes— many people are sensitive to the acid in this fruit/vegetable); toasted sunflower seeds; chopped olives or avocado; marinated artichoke hearts or cold vegetables from last night's dinner; chunks of cold chicken, turkey, salmon, beef, or lamb. If you're not allergic, try adding beans (garbanzos are delicious) or tofu. On occasion, I'll add canned salmon. Canned tuna can become an allergy because people consume it so frequently. Fresh tuna, on the other hand, is usually non-allergic, since it's rarely eaten.

- Consider sprinkling the top of your salad with goat feta cheese, or sheep cheddar or Romano cheese. Products made from cows' milk cause me to experience fluid retention, puffy eyes, blocked eustachian tubes, postnasal drip, and mild deafness in my left ear. Because sheep and goat products belong to a different food family, they usually don't trigger histamine reactions in dairy-sensitive people. As I've said before, butter is a dairy product, but usually permissible, since it contains very few milk solids, which is what can trigger immune reactions.

- Make roll-ups for a quick and savory meal. Simply place some protein in a large lettuce or cabbage leaf, and roll it up. Roll-ups can be made more exotic by adding any of the vegetables or ingredients from the list above; or try using thinly sliced pieces of ham or turkey for a tasty change-of-pace. (Wasa crackers also make a nice addition to lunch, but I usually stay away from carbohydrates with this meal also—I find that I have better energy that way).

Dressings

- Partake in any oil and vinegar dressing. Even if you're eradicating candida and ferments should be avoided, vinegar in small amounts should be okay. Just watch if you start having nasal congestion, a runny nose, postnasal drip, or headaches, as these are signs of ferment-sensitivity.

- For the first 30 days of your program, stay away from dressings containing sugar and dairy products—*read labels.* Add mayonnaise to your dressing to make it creamy. (Mayonnaise is made from eggs and oil, and doesn't contain dairy products.) People who aren't sensitive to citrus fruits (lemon, orange, and grapefruit) may use lemon or lime juice in place of vinegar in salad dressings.

- Try this dressing, which I make when I'm at home:

    > 3 Tbsp. flaxseed (high in essential fatty acids) or olive oil
    > 1 tsp. vinegar—apple cider, balsamic, or rice wine variety
    > ½ tsp. creamy Dijon mustard (in place of Dijon mustard, I use fresh herbs, such as chopped basil, dill, or parsley)
    > A pinch of coarse Celtic sea salt
    > Fresh ground pepper
    > Shake well in a glass jar and serve over salad

- For something different, I use sesame seeds, fresh ginger, and one tsp soy sauce or soy sauce alternative.

Mid-Afternoon Snack

- Eat a handful of roasted, unsalted nuts with a cup of herbal tea. (If you're allergic to nuts, substitute another protein. Also remember that nuts often contain mold, so if you have a mold sensitivity, be aware.) Be sure that the nuts are roasted. I roast them myself by placing them on a cookie sheet in an oven preheated to 250–300 degrees for approximately ½ hour or until golden brown. Nothing's more delicious than a pan of freshly roasted nuts, and this protein snack boosts my energy and sustains me until dinner.

- Spread almond, cashew, hazelnut, or macadamia nut butter on top of whole rye crackers, rice cakes or crackers (found in the oriental foods section of most grocery stores). Remember that peanuts are legumes, which is a common allergy. Seed butters are also tasty on crackers. Once again, wash down your snack with a cup of herbal tea with natural sweetener.

- Dip ½ of a thinly sliced apple in nut or seed butter. (Keep in mind that carbohydrate grams in fruit add up quickly: ½ apple contains eight grams of carbohydrate.)

- Fill two celery stalks with almond or cashew nut butter.

- Roll two ham, beef, or salami slices around a chunk of cucumber or a hunk of goat feta or sheep cheddar cheese.

- Enjoy two deviled eggs.

Soups

- People are always asking me for my soup recipes. My mother, a dietician, was a fabulous soup maker, and I learned from her that a soup could be made from any combination of ingredients that you have on hand, built around a stock and seasoned to taste. On many a winter evening, our family would sit down to a healthy and delicious meal of one of my mother's famous soups and a loaf of her homemade bread.

- When a body is sick or in a weakened state, nurturing soups, which are easy to digest, can provide a welcome change from solid food. Chicken soup and broth are well-known healing elixirs, but many people overlook the benefits of naturally occurring iron, B vitamins, and nutritious marrow, found in beef meat and bones. Following is my recipe for beef broth, which has been useful for many of my clients.

Caroline's Beef Broth

- Take a large bag of beef bones. Choose bones with some meat left on them—beef ribs or rib bones would work nicely.

- Put the bones on a baking sheet or in a shallow roasting pan and bake at 300 degrees for about two hours. This removes the fat and enhances the flavor of the brew.

- Remove the bones from the oven and boil on a low simmer for another two hours.

- For added flavor, add a chopped onion or carrot to the roasting bones. These can be boiled in the pot with the bones. (Be sure you are aware of onion sensitivities before adding them to the mixture.) Salt may be added to the broth if tolerated and desired.

- Strain and drink the broth. Drink as much as you desire—when people are weak or very ill, I recommend approximately four to six cups per day.

- The broth may also be consumed as a beverage, along with regular meals.

Dinner

- Eat any vegetable, cooked or raw, and any animal or vegetable protein source to which you're not allergic. (I find that most CNS people do better and feel more stable with animal protein.) Muscle test or use a pendulum to hone your intuition and determine your best protein choices. Along with your protein and vegetable choice, add any non-allergic source of carbohydrates. If you're trying to lose weight, keep an eye on your carbohydrates grams. Remember that one medium potato, one cup cooked rice, and one ear of corn all contain 20 grams of carbohydrates.

- Many people who have poor absorption through the gastrointestinal tract or stomach problems don't seem to tolerate grains well. To give the digestive system a rest, try using starchy vegetables, such as squash, sweet potatoes, or yams in place of grains for a few weeks. You'll instinctively know whether grains or the starchy vegetables are easier for you to digest. I usually have squash (yellow winter, butternut, or Danish) with my dinner.

- Eat slowly and *enjoy* your meal. Treat yourself to a beautiful table setting and pleasant surroundings while eating. Also teach your children how to respect their bodies and eat in this way.

- Wait 20 minutes after your meal to allow the "feel-good" brain chemical serotonin to be released. Most people won't feel hungry after such a meal, but after 20 minutes, if you still are, go back and have *more dinner*—don't just reflexively grab some dessert.

- After dinner, brew a cup of herbal tea, coffee substitute, or decaffeinated coffee, unless you're legume sensitive (coffee is a legume). Drink it unsweetened, or if you need that sweet taste, add a drop of natural sweetener, available at health-food stores. Often just the very taste of a sweetener, even a natural one, can evoke a need for *more* sweet!

Desserts

- One choice for an after-dinner snack could be ⅓ of a high-protein, low-carbohydrate bar purchased from a health-food store. Be careful though, as many of these bars contain ingredients to which you might be allergic, such as whey (found in dairy products), cocoa or peanuts (beans/legumes), as well as additives and chemicals. For most people, ⅛ of a bar shouldn't trigger reactions, but research this for yourself. I'm not a big fan of these bars. I feel that, for the most part, they're for emergency use only, such as when you're on a long hike, stuck in an airport or stranded at the side of a road. But for many people, the transition away from sugar is very difficult, and some allowable sweets become an important lifeline. Fresh fruit can also be a welcome after-dinner choice, but the best pick is no dessert at all.

- I reserve desserts for the times when I'm having dinner out with friends and something homemade or very special will tempt me. Usually after such an exposure I'll feel "off," tired, or have that hungover feeling the next day. When I'm working or speaking, dessert is not worth the price my body has to pay. If every treat represents $100 in life-force energy, I need to be careful where and how I spend it.

- If you're disciplined, and a small amount of sweet won't derail your program, try a rice flour cookie or a piece of coconut pecan crunch. Here are some recipes for you to experiment with. (Though both of these recipes use honey, the amount in one serving is so small that it won't affect a candida-eradication program.)

Rice Flour Birds' Nest Cookies

(Makes about two dozen cookies;
about 15 grams of carbohydrate per cookie.)

Ingredients:

1½ cups of rice flour
½ cup tapioca starch (available in Asian
   food stores)
¼ tsp. baking powder
¼ tsp. salt
1 cup butter
2 Tbsp. honey or 1½ tsp. Stevia or other
   natural sweetener

Garnishes (optional)
¼ cup shredded unsweetened coconut
2 Tbsp. all-fruit jam
Walnuts, cashews, or filberts

- Preheat oven to 350 degrees. Cream butter and dry ingredients until well mixed.

- Add the vanilla and honey; chill mixture in fridge for approximately ½ hour.

- Form into balls and press one side of the "ball" into unsweetened coconut.

- Pat onto greased cookie sheet—with the coconut side facing up—and make a small well in middle of each cookie.

- Drop ¼ tsp all-fruit jam in the center, or add a nut piece in the center.

- Bake 20 minutes. Cool well in the fridge, then carefully transfer to cookie tin and store in the freezer. Take out one at a time (don't thaw) and enjoy after dinner with a cup of herbal tea.

Coconut Pecan Crunch

(Makes about two dozen treats; low carbohydrate—approx. 8 grams per 1-inch square.)

Ingredients:

1 cup butter
2 Tbsp. honey or 1 tsp. Stevia to taste
1 tsp. pure vanilla extract
3 Tbsp. powdered carob
½ to 1 cup toasted pecans, walnuts, or a
    mixture of favorite nuts
¼ cup shredded unsweetened coconut

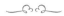

- Grease a 9" square baking pan or pie plate. Line the bottom with roasted nuts and coconut.

- Melt butter over very low heat; add honey, vanilla, and carob. Pour this mixture over the nuts and coconut.

- Place directly in the freezer (this treat needs to be stored frozen.) In approximately ½ hour, when solid, cut and serve. Enjoy one piece after dinner, with a cup of herbal tea.

- This treat isn't suitable for people who have nut allergies or are sensitive to some varieties of beans.

Options . . .

This way of eating is never boring. Try to treat yourself like royalty by choosing wholesome, even expensive ingredients. (Actually your food bill will probably decline when you're not purchasing expensive packaged items.) Use olive oil when sautéing vegetables or meats. Try cold marinated vegetables as a change from, or an addition to, salads. Save leftover vegetables and add them to a morning omelette. Experiment with fresh ginger, herbs, and spices. Treat yourself well, and *cook!* Some people actually will find themselves cooking for the first time.

I remember consulting with a woman who lived in Los Angeles, which is famous for its glitz, glamour, and fancy restaurants. When I broached the subject of cooking to her, she was horrified, exclaiming that she never cooked, but purchased all her meals and beverages in restaurants. When I asked her if she had a stove, she paused for a moment and admitted that, although she'd lived in her current residence for five years, she'd never once used the stove!

For people like these, I recommend the use of a slow cooker or tabletop grill. A slow cooker works very well and is a lazy way to prepare an evening meal—eight hours ahead of time, in the morning.

Using a Slow Cooker or Tabletop Grill

- Choose any sort of meat you wish to cook—chicken, turkey, or beef works well, and lamb shanks are especially tasty cooked in a slow cooker. Place the meat inside, and add approximately two cups of water, stock, chicken or beef broth. Add a diced onion, two chopped celery stalks, a cut-up carrot, and season to taste with salt, pepper, fresh herbs, or nonfermented soy sauce.

- Turn on the slow cooker and leave it to simmer for the day. Eight hours later, you'll return to delicious smells and an inviting meal. Cook a pot of rice or a baked potato, fix a quick salad, and voilà! The evening meal is prepared, and there are plenty of leftovers.

- Another convenient way to cook is with a tabletop grill, which is about the size of a tennis racquet and sits at an angle on the kitchen counter so that fat from the meat drips down into a container below the grill.

- Place any meat you wish to cook on the surface of the hot grill—chicken breasts, turkey sausages, steak, or lamb chops work well. Brush the surface of the meat with nonfermented soy sauce, and sprinkle with herbs or spices. Then arrange cut-up vegetables next to the meat— eggplant slices, zucchini strips, or peppers, for example. After 10 to 15 minutes, turn the meat over and grill the other side.

- Remove the vegetables. Serve the meal with any appropriate starch or carbohydrate of your choice.

The body knows that it's loved. As you prepare your foods with love and consciousness, this energy is positively transmitted to body parts and processes.

Eating Out

- Eating in restaurants doesn't need to be difficult. If you're sensitive to wheat, you can always order rice or a baked potato with dinner, or home fries or hash browns in place of toast at breakfast.

- Salads are usually available, as are steamed vegetables—order them without cheese or sauce, as many sauces contain dairy products. Order a vinaigrette for salad dressing, or just use plain oil and vinegar. This way, you'll be avoiding dressings that contain dairy products. Ask about the ingredients of sauces and dressings. If in doubt, order it "on the side," and trust your instincts regarding amounts to take.

- Salad bars can be a marvelous choice since you get to control your own portions and choices.

- Eggs, chicken, turkey, fish, shellfish, lamb, beef, pork, beans, and legumes are all good protein choices. Some forms of animal protein are more digestible than others. Learn to muscle-test, or use a pendulum to determine appropriate choices.

- Personally, I rarely eat beans, which upset my digestive system and give me gas—not great when working with the public. Although high in protein and well tolerated by many people, beans are also high in carbohydrates.

- Tofu is made from soybeans. Soy can increase estrogen levels, and high estrogen levels have been linked to breast cancer. I'm in the middle of my menopause years, and recently my estrogen levels were tested and found to be quite high; therefore, I hardly ever eat tofu or consume any soy products. In addition, tofu is rarely found on restaurant menus unless you're in a vegetarian or Asian restaurant.

- For a beverage choice that won't upset your plan, carry a bag of herbal tea with you. Most restaurants will bring you a mug of hot water in which to make your favorite brew.

Traveling

- I always carry nuts (usually roasted almonds) with me when I travel. I also try to carry a selection of protein bars. These can be a lifesaver if a flight is delayed or I arrive at a hotel late at night and I'm ravenous. I rarely can eat any food on an airplane—I'll pick away at what's offered and fill in with nuts. I'll often carry cold meat slices in a small insulated bag, which, for obvious reasons, need to be consumed within several hours of leaving home.

- I carry a package of Ry Krisp or Wasa crackers with me at all times—in this way, I can avoid wheat and its subsequent ill effects at all times. I also carry a small, plastic, screw-top container of cashew or almond butter, sealed in a plastic bag, which I liberally coat on the crackers for a fast and nutritious breakfast or late-night snack.

- I like to choose hotels with a refrigerator in my room. I'll ask a friend in the city I'm visiting to stock the refrigerator ahead of time, with a selection of vegetables, hard-boiled eggs, and cold meats and poultry. I draw from this supply while I'm working during the day, and then I usually enjoy dinner with friends or a restaurant meal at night.

- When I'm exposed to sweet desserts, I use my intuition and ask how many bites I should take before my body will react from any ill effects. The answer might be two bites, or ten— depending on the item. After the intuited number of bites are consumed, I simply put down my fork, because if I go "over the line," I'll invariably feel off the next day.

- I'm acutely aware of my limits with wine; therefore, I drink it very occasionally—probably only once or twice a month on average. I approach the glass of wine in the same way as a dessert, tuning in to the beverage and sensing the amount that would be "enough." I find that about six sips is my limit. Because I'm a CNS type, and wine is a powerful stimulant, a small amount will change my body chemistry and alter my personality. But on occasion, I like the buzz that wine gives me, along with its relaxing effects. I also find I get less dehydrated if I take one sip of wine and then four sips of water, alternating in this manner until my designated number of sips is finished. Then I look at the glass of wine and know that it's time to switch to sparkling water with a slice of lemon or lime. With this approach, I tolerate these items in small amounts.

Discipline in food consumption is an important level of personal mastery. Foods are chemicals and medicines. When we feel good physically, there benefits are felt on the emotional and spiritual levels as well.

When you're starting a food program, keep everything as simple as possible. Don't try to get fancy or complicated, like trying to make intricate sauces out of alternative and exotic types of flour. Avoid the sauces and the strain on yourself, and within 30 days enjoy the occasional sauce in a restaurant or at a friend's home.

This isn't the time to be making angel food cakes out of mung bean flour. You'll be back to eating *real* angel food cake on an occasional basis after you've spent just a few weeks clearing your body of toxins and histamine reactions. If you're preparing meals for a family, cook normally for them and stick to your program. Enjoy yourself—this is a life- and health-changing experience.

Food Families

The following is a list of common food families. When avoiding offending foods, it can be helpful to check the food family list and avoid foods that are in the same family. *Single food families.*

PLANTS

Apple
Apple
Apple Cider
Pear
Pectin
Quince & Seed
Vinegar

Bamboo shoots*

Banana
Arrowroot
Banana
Plantain

Barley
Malt

Beet
Beet
Beet Sugar
Chard
Lamb's-quarter

Spinach
Thistle

Birch
Filbert
Hazelnut
Wintergreen

Brazil nut*

Buckwheat
Buckwheat
Garden sorrel
Rhubarb

Cacao
Cocoa bean
Cocoa chocolate
Kola nut

Cactus
Cactus
Prickly pear
Tequila

Cane
Sugar
Molasses

Caper*

Carrot
Carrots
Celeriac
Celery
Coriander
Cumin
Dill
Fennel
Parsley
Parsnip

Cashew
Cashew
Mango
Pistachio

Chicory*

Citrus
Angostura
Citron
Grapefruit
Kumquat
Lemon
Lime
Orange
Tangerine

Composite
Artichoke

Dandelion
Endive
Escarole
Jerusalem artichoke
Lettuce
Sesame oil
Sesame seed
Sunflower oil
Sunflower seed

Corn
Dextrose (Glucose)
Meal
Oil
Starch
Sugar
Syrup

Ebony
Persimmon

Fungi
Baker's yeast
Brewer's yeast
Mold
Mushroom

Ginger
Cardamom
Ginger
Turmeric

Gooseberry
Currant
Gooseberry

Gourd
Casaba
Cantaloupe
Cucumber
Gherkin
Honeydew
Muskmelon
Persian melon
Pumpkin
Squash
Watermelon

Grape
Brandy
Champagne
Cream of tartar
Grapes
Raisin
Wine
Wine vinegar

Heath
Blueberry
Cranberry
Huckleberry

Iris
Saffron

Laurel
Avocado
Bay leaves
Cinnamon
Sassafras

Lily
Aloes
Asparagus
Chives
Garlic
Leek
Onion
Sarsaparilla

Legumes
Black-eyed pea
Carob
Green pea
Jack bean
Kidney bean
Lecithin
Lentil
Licorice
Lima bean
Navy bean
Peanut
Peanut oil
Pinto
Senna
Soybean
Soy oil
Soy flour
String bean
Tonka bean

Madder*
Coffee bean

Mallow
Cottonseed meal

Cottonseed oil
Okra (Gumbo)

Maple
Maple sugar
Maple syrup

Millet*

Mint
Basil
Horehound
Marjoram
Mint
Oregano
Peppermint
Sage
Spearmint
Thyme

Morning Glory
Sweet potato
Yam

Mulberry
Breadfruit
Fig
Hop
Mulberry

Mustard
Broccoli
Cabbage
Cauliflower
Chinese cabbage

Collard
Horseradish
Kale
Kohlrabi
Kraut
Mustard
Mustard greens
Mustard seeds
Radish
Rape (canola)
Rutabaga
Sprouts
Turnips
Watercress

Myrtle
Allspice
Cloves
Guava
Paprika
Pimento

Nightshade
Belladonna
Black pepper
Chili pepper
Eggplant
Green pepper
Potato
Red capsicum
Red cayenne
Red pepper
Tobacco
Tomato
White pepper

Nutmeg
Mace
Nutmeg

Oak
Acorn
Chestnut

Oats*

Olive
Black olives
Green olives
Olive oil

Orchid*
Vanilla

Palm
Coconut
Date
Palm cabbage
Sago

Parsley
Anise
Angelica
Caraway
Celery
Celery seed
Carrots
Celeriac
Coriander
Cumin
Dill
Fennel

Parsley
Parsnips

Pawpaw
Pawpaw
Papain
Papaya

Pine
Juniper
Pinion nut

Pineapple*

Pomegranate*

Poppy*
Poppy seeds

Plum
Almond
Apricot
Cherry
Nectarine
Peach
Plum
Prune
Wild cherry

Rice*

Rye*

Rose
Blackberry
Boysenberry

Dewberry
Loganberry
Raspberry
Strawberry
Youngberry

Soapberry
Lichi nut

Tapioca*

Tea*

Walnut
Black walnut
English walnut
Hickory nut
Pecan

Wheat
Bran
Farina
Flour
Gluten flour
Wheat germ
Whole wheat

Wild Rice*

MEATS

Butter
Cheese
Gelatin

Poultry
Chicken
Chicken eggs
Duck
Duck eggs
Goose
Goose eggs
Guinea hen
Grouse
Partridge
Pheasant
Squab
Turkey
Turkey eggs

Mammals
Beef
  • Butter
  • Cheese
  • Gelatin
  • Milk
  • Veal
Buffalo
Goat
  • Milk
  • Cheese
  • Mutton
Lamb
Pork
  • Bacon
  • Ham
Rabbit
Venison

Fish*

Crustaceans
Crab
Crayfish
Lobster
Shrimp

Mollusks
Abalone
Clam
Mussel
Oyster
Scallop
Snail
Squid

Hidden Food Sources

You may be surprised to find that your favorite foods are hiding out in the most unlikely places. This list can help you to identify offending foods, which could be hidden in other products. Read labels and get to know the ingredients of common, combination foods.

Corn
All baked goods
Aspirin
Baking powder
Beer, ales
Biscuits
Breads, pastries
Butter substitute
Cakes, cookies
Candies
Carbonated beverages
Chewing gum
Cornmeal
Corn oil
Cough syrups
Cream pies
Cured hams
Custard
Doughnuts
Graham crackers
Gravies
Grits
Gummed papers
Instant teas

Ketchup
Margarine
Non-dairy creamers
Pancake mix
Pie crusts
Popcorn
Puddings, instant
Salad dressings
Sandwich spreads
Sausages
Soups, creamed
Stamp glue
Starch
Toothpaste
Tortillas
Whiskey

Egg
Baking powders
Bavarian cream
Breaded foods
Breads
Cake flours
Cakes

Custards
Eggs
French toast
Fritters
Frostings
Frying batters
Griddle cakes
Hamburger patties
Hollandaise sauce
Ice cream
Icings
Macaroni
Macaroons
Marshmallows
Mayonnaise
Meat loaf
Meringues
Noodles
Pancakes
Puddings
Rolls
Salad dressings
Sauces
Sausages
Soufflés
Waffles

Milk
Biscuits
Breads
Buttermilk
Cakes
Cheese
Cheese dishes
Chocolate milk
Chowders
Cookies

Creamed foods
Custards
Fritters
Gravies
Ice cream
Malted cocoa
Mashed potatoes
Omelettes
Ovaltine
Pancakes
Pancake mix
Potatoes, scalloped
Powdered milk
Salad dressing, creamy
Sherbets
Soda crackers
Soufflés
Soups, creamed
Sour cream
Waffles
Whey
Yogurt

Soybeans
Asian sauces
Baby foods
Biscuits
Breads
Butter substitute
Cakes
Cereals
Cooking spray
Crackers
Hard candies
Ice cream
Lecithin
Lunch meats

Margarine
Mayonnaise
Milk substitute
Oils
Pastries
Salad dressings
Soups
Soy flour
Soy noodles
Tempura
Textured vegetable protein
Tofu

Wheat
Bagels
Biscuits
Bologna
Bread
Breaded meats/fish
Cakes
Cereals
Cookies
Corn bread
Crackers
Doughnuts
Dumplings
Flour
Gravies
Hot cakes
Liverwurst
Lunch meats
Macaroni
Pasta
Pie crust

Yeast
Beer
Bovril
Brandy
Breads
Buns
Cakes
Cereals
Cheeses
Chocolate
Condiments
Cookies
Crackers
French dressing
Fruit juices
Gin
Horseradish
Malted milk
Mayonnaise
Olives
Pastries
Pickles
Pretzels
Rolls
Rum
Sauerkraut
Soy sauce
Tomato sauce
Truffles
Vinegar
Vitamins
Vodka
Whiskey
Wine

Food Families and Hidden Food Sources lists, adapted and used with permission: Dr. Julian N. Kenyon, Dove Clinic for Integrated Medicine, 97 Harley Street, London, U.K. www.doveclinic.com.

Sample Carbohydrate Grams

Food	Amount	Carbohydrate Grams
Animal Protein		
Chicken, Beef, Fish, Lamb, Turkey, Veal, Pork (Ham, Bacon), Shellfish, Wild Meats, Eggs	any amount	0
Dairy Products		
Whole milk	1 cup	12
Ice cream	½ cup	15
Cheese	1 oz. hard	1
Cottage cheese	½ cup	4
Sour cream	1 Tbsp.	1
Yogurt	½ cup	8
Fats		
Butter	1 Tbsp.	0
French dressing	1 Tbsp.	2
Vegetable oil	unlimited	0
Olive oil	unlimited	0
Mayonnaise	1 Tbsp.	0
Nuts		
Mixed	¼ cup	5
Almonds	¼ cup	5
Peanut butter	2 Tbsp.	5
Cashew nut butter	2 Tbsp.	11

Vegetables

Alfalfa sprouts (raw)	½ cup	0
Arugula	unlimited	0
Artichoke	1 medium	14
Asparagus	10 spears	4
Beans, green	1 cup cooked	8
Beets	1 cup cooked	6
Broccoli	1 cup cooked	5
Brussels sprouts	6	5
Cabbage	1 cup shredded, raw	3
Cabbage	1 cup cooked	5
Carrots	1 medium, raw	5
Carrots	1 cup cooked	12
Cauliflower	1 cup	4
Celery	2 stalks	2
Corn	1 ear	20
Cucumber	1 medium	6
Eggplant	1 cup cooked	6
Kale	1 cup cooked	3
Lettuce	unlimited	0
Okra	1 cup	11
Onions	½ cup, raw	5
Onions	½ cup cooked	10
Green peas	1 cup	20
Green pepper	1 large	5
Potatoes	1 small	20
Spinach	1 cup cooked	4
Squash	1 cup cooked	10
Tomatoes	1 medium	4
Turnip	½ cup	8
Ketchup	1 Tbsp.	5
Tomato juice	1 cup	5

Beans (Legumes)		
Tofu	½ cup	20
Lima beans	½ cup	25
Kidney beans	½ cup	13
White beans	½ cup	22
Fava beans	½ cup	16
Soy flour	½ cup	12
Fruit		
Apples	1 large	20
Apricots	4 small	14
Avocados	½ medium	5
Bananas	1 medium	25
Strawberries	1 cup	7
Raspberries	1 cup	8
Blackberries	1 cup	10
Blueberries	1 cup	17
Cantaloupe	1 cup	12
Grapefruit	½ small	8
Grapes	½ cup	8
Lemons	1 medium	8
Limes	1 medium	8
Oranges	1 small	11
Orange juice	1 cup	22
Peaches	1 medium	8
Pears	1 medium	20
Pineapple	1 cup	17
Pineapple	½ cup, canned	18
Plums	1 large	18
Watermelon	1 cup	11
Breads and Cereals		
Bagel	1	27
Bread	1 slice	20
Hamburger bun	1	23

English muffin	1	25
Pita round	1	20
Rice cake	1	8
Rice crackers	2	4
Saltine cracker	1	2
Wasa (rye) cracker	1	7
Cornflakes	1 cup	17
Oatmeal	1 cup cooked	20
Shredded wheat	1 large	23
Spaghetti, macaroni, pasta	1 cup	25
Noodles (egg)	1 cup	26
Rice	1 cup cooked	20
Sweeteners		
Honey	1 Tbsp.	15
White sugar	1 tsp.	4
Brown sugar	1 Tbsp.	10
Stevia (herb sweetener)	1 tsp.	1
Syrup	1 Tbsp.	15
Spirits		
Wine (red or white)	1 glass	3
Light Beer	8 oz.	4

For a complete list of carbohydrate grams refer to *Protein Power*, Eades (Bantam, 1999).

Common Allergens— and Where They're Located

Algae: stagnant water, fish tanks, swimming pools, lakes, freshwater swamps, trapped fresh water areas

Candida albicans: species of yeast common to all humans

Chalk: blackboard chalk, drywall, plaster dust

Dust mites: bedding, carpets, and mattresses

Feathers: pillows, quilts, and sleeping bags; parkas; in household, farm, and wild birds

Grain dust: animal feeds, grain storage

Grasses: cultivated lawn and wild grasses

House dust: bedding, fibers, and carpets in all areas of the home (house dust can contain dust mite feces)

Scotch broom pollen: yellow flowering bush found in coastal areas

Tree pollens (deciduous): alder, ash, beech, birch, elm, oak, hazel, hickory, poplar, maple, Scotch sycamore, walnut, willow

Tree pollens (evergreen): balsam, cedar, fir, hemlock, pine, spruce, redwood

Weed pollens: alfalfa, dandelion, clover, dock, lamb's-quarter, pigweed, ragweed, sagebrush

Wood dust: sawdust and wood shavings

Wool: wool clothing and woven wool fabrics

Molds

Molds, a natural part of the life cycle of all decaying plant and food materials, thrive in dark and damp areas. Mold spores are prevalent in the air in damp climates, and mildew is sometimes incorrectly called mold. Most common foods, fresh and prepared, contain a variety of molds. Following is a list of the different strains of mold and where they can be found.

Acremonium: soil, damp paper, fabric dust, wood by-products

Alternaria, Epicoccum, Sporobolomyces: decomposing plants, moldy vegetables and fruits

Aspergillus: composts, hay, damp vegetation, damp fabric, leather, grains, fruits, soy sauce, cheeses, corn, peanuts

Botrytis: moldy fruits, grapes, some flowers

Cryptococcus: pigeons, pigeon feces, dust in outside air, indoor and outdoor plants

Fusarium: vegetables, beans, cabbage, corn, peas, sweet potatoes, squashes, tomatoes, whole grains and flours, decaying plants and houseplants

Hormodendrum: leaves, rotting plants, decaying trees, rotting wood, leftover foods; appears as black specks on windows, dank walls and corners, and damp stored clothing

Mucor: farming areas, animal waste, soil

Penicillium: on fruits, breads, cheese, the surface of jams and condiments, damp shoes and clothing; common bread mold is used in the production of penicillin

Phoma: paper, damp books and magazines

Pullularia: decaying plants and soil

Rhodotorula: a common mold existing in the air and soil

Stachy Botrys: dark, black mold, which, in addition to being an allergen, may also contain mycotoxins; thrives on damp, high cellulose, low-nitrogen containing material such as: wall board, paper, fabrics and carpet backing (resulting from water damage)

Streptomyces: basements, potatoes, plants, plant undergrowth

Trichoderma: damp basements, damp fabrics, forest growth

Adapted and used with permission of Russell B. Olinsky, M.Sc., Enviro-Health, 77 West Coolidge St., #132, Phoenix, AZ 85013, (602) 432-1449.

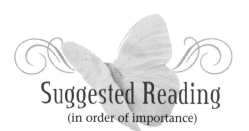

Suggested Reading
(in order of importance)

The Yeast Connection Handbook, by William Crook, M.D.

Protein Power, by Michael and Mary Dan Eades, M.D.

The Missing Diagnosis, by Orian Truss, M.D.

Is This Your Child? Discovering and Treating Unrecognized Allergies in Adults and Children, by Doris Rapp, M.D.

Is This Your Child's World?, by Doris Rapp, M.D.

Environmentally Sick Schools (Video), by Doris Rapp, M.D.

Dr. Crook Discusses Alternatives to Ritalin in the Management of ADHD, by William Crook, M.D.

Molecules of Emotion, by Candace Pert, Ph.D.

Heal Your Body, by Louise L. Hay

You Can Heal Your Life, by Louise L. Hay

Pinpoint Your Destiny: Discover Passion, Purpose, and Calling By Using Your Natural Talents, by Curtis Adney

The Twelve Conditions of a Miracle: The Miracle Worker's Handbook, by Dr. Michael Abrams

Prayer and the Five Stages of Healing, by Ron Roth, Ph.D.

The Heart's Wisdom: A Practical Guide to Growing Through Love, by Joyce and Barry Vissel, M.D.

A Flash of Lightning in the Dark of Night: A Guide to the Bodhisattva's Way of Life, by The Dalai Lama

Anatomy of the Spirit, by Caroline Myss, Ph.D.

Why People Don't Heal and How They Can, by Caroline Myss, Ph.D.

Closer to the Light, by Melvin Morse, M.D.

How to Know God, by Deepak Chopra, M.D.

Embracing the Beloved, by Ondrea Levine and Stephen Levine, M.D.

Healing Yourself: A Step-by-Step Program for Better Health Through Imagery, by Martin Rossman, M.D.

Prayer Is Good Medicine, by Larry Dossey, M.D.

Your Hidden Food Allergies Are Making You Fat: The ALCAT Food Sensitivities Weight Loss Breakthrough, by Rudy Rivera M.D., and Roger D. Deutsch

What Your Doctor May Not Tell You about Menopause, by John Lee, M.D.

Words to Love By, by Mother Teresa

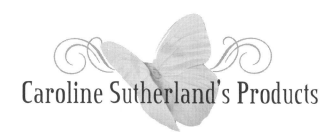

Caroline Sutherland's Products

Sleep Talking® Tapes for Adults & Children.
(All per-item prices include shipping and handling.)

Couples/Serenity & Tranquility
This tape works to remove blocks to a loving, healthy relationship. In a few short weeks, experience a deeper level of joy and bonding—with your loved one and with yourself. Soothing wave background.
For adults • 60 mins. • $13

Body Alive/Deep Relaxation and Sleep
You're guided through a series of phrases about health, immunity, weight, and abundant energy. The soothing, positive wave sounds help to improve sleep as well—this is a great tape for insomniacs.
For adults • 60 mins. • $13

Letting Go of the Past/Moving Forward
Have you ever felt unable to let go of the past? Release old resentments and grievances with soothing reassurances, repeated nightly. Caroline's restful, encouraging voice gives you the confidence to move forward, and the willingness to let go. Soothing wave background.
For adults • 60 mins. • $13

Beautiful & Ageless
Deep relaxation and positive programming for women in all phases of menopause—this tape really helps with personal motivation, anxiety, and sleeplessness. Soothing wave - background.
For adults • 60 mins. • $13

Overcoming Jet Lag & Travel Fatigue
A very effective tape, recommended by travelers, flight attendants, pilots, and business people for jet lag and fear of flying. Soothing wave background.
For adults • 60 mins. • $13

Meditation & Music
A relaxing guided-meditation tape designed to center you, focus your breath, work with your own affirmations, and help to access that deep state of peace within you. This tape is set to beautiful music created by award-winning musician Paul Armitage.
For adults • 60 mins. • $13

Motivation & Confidence for Teenagers and Young People
Parents say this tape can put the "terrific" back into your teenager. In three to four weeks of nightly listening, teenagers can expect to feel an increase in self-esteem, motivation, and positive choices. Soothing wave background.
For adolescents (ages 12 and up) • 60 mins. • $13

Ace Those Exams
Decreases the fear and anxiety of exams, while increasing memory and mental ability—it really works! For teens and adults. Soothing wave background.
For adults and adolescents (ages 12 and up) • 60 mins. • $13

Body Alive (Children)/Confidence & Self-Esteem
Helps your child to understand the body processes, as well as developing a healthy attitude about food choices, physical activity, confidence, and positive values. Set to beautiful music.
For children ages 3–10 • 60 mins. • $13

Schoolwork & Making Friends
Helps to develop love and excitement about school and learning—also helps the child to overcome blocks and barriers to playing and sharing with others. Set to enchanting music.
For children ages 3–10 • 60 mins. • $13

Mommy, I Hurt . . . Mommy, I Love You
A self-help guide for parents and children. This 65-page book inspires parents to help their children over the "rough spots" in a unique, reassuring way. Uses the principles of relaxation therapy and creative visualization.
4" x 6" • $10

The Heart of the Family
This parent-education video covering a variety of topics shows unique ways to strengthen communication between parent and child and blended family members.
2 hrs. • $22

—⟡⟡—

My Little Angel® Products

Welcome to the world of *My Little Angel*—angels, audiotapes, and story books that reassure and encourage children.

All sets include a soft, cuddly angel, which is available in either white or ethnic (brown) faces, and is great for both boys and girls. Each angel is handmade and machine washable in soft, cotton velour. Also included is a positive, uplifting 60-minute story/music audiotape. (Visit **www.angels4kids.com**.)

My Little Angel Tells Me I'm Special®. The story helps children to fall asleep and build self-esteem. A general tape useful for all children—from babies to ten years of age. (Adults and teens love it, too.)

My Little Angel Helps Me and My Family®. The story supports and comforts children who are adjusting to a family breakup, separation, or divorce.

My Little Angel Helps Me in the Hospital®. The story calms, comforts, and reassures children who require hospitalization for major or minor surgery, serious illness, cancer treatment, burns, or any surgical procedure.

My Little Angel Loves Me®. The story reassures, comforts and supports children (and adults) who have been abused, traumatized, or mistreated.

ALL SETS COST $29.95 (U.S.)
PRICES INCLUDE SHIPPING AND HANDLING
Prices subject to change without notice

For a complete listing of all of Caroline Sutherland's products, seminars, assessments, and trainings, write to:

Sutherland Communications Inc.
Caroline M. Sutherland
816 Peace Portal Drive, PMB 199
Blaine, WA 98230
or
visit Caroline on-line at:
www.carolinesutherland.com
or
www.angels4kids.com

Self-Help Resources

The following list of resources can be used to access information on a variety of issues. The addresses and telephone numbers listed are for the national headquarters; look in your local yellow pages under "Community Services" for resources closer to your area.

In addition to the following groups, other self-help organizations may be available in your area to assist your healing and recovery for a particular life crisis not listed here. Consult your telephone directory, call a counseling center or help line near you, or contact:

AIDS

CBC National AIDS Hotline
(800) 342-2437

Children with AIDS (CWA) Project of America
(800) 866-AIDS (24-hour hotline)

The Names Project —AIDS Quilt
(800) 872-6263

Project Inform
19655 Market St., Ste. 220
San Francisco, CA 94103
(415) 558-8669

PWA Coalition
50 W. 17th St.
New York, NY 10011

Spanish HIV/STD/AIDS Hotline
(800) 344-7432

TTY (Hearing Impaired) AIDS Hotline (CDC National HIV/AIDS)
(800) 243-7889

ALCOHOL ABUSE

Al-Anon Family Headquarters
1600 Corporate Landing
Parkway

Virginia Beach, VA
23454-5617
(800) 4AL-ANON

**Alcoholics Anonymous
(AA)**
General Service Office
475 Riverside Dr.
New York, NY 10115
(212) 870-3400

**Children of Alcoholics
Foundation**
164 W. 74th St.
New York, NY 10023
(800) 359-COAF

Meridian Council, Inc.
Administrative Offices
4 Elmcrest Terrace
Norwalk, CT 06850

**Mothers Against Drunk
Driving (MADD)**
(254) 690-6233

**National Association of
Children of Alcoholics
(NACOA)**
11426 Rockville Pike,
Ste. 100
Rockville, MD 20852
(301) 468-0985
(888) 554-2627

**National Clearinghouse
for Alcohol and Drug
Information (NCADI)**
P.O. Box 234
Rockville, MD 20852
(301) 468-2600

**National Council on
Alcoholism and Drug
Dependence (NCADD)**
12 West 21st St.
New York, NY 10010
(212) 206-6770
(800) 475-HOPE

Women for Sobriety
(800) 333-1606

ALZHEIMER'S DISEASE

Alzheimer's Association
919 N. Michigan Ave.,
Ste. 1100
Chicago, IL 60611
(800) 621-0379
www.alz.org

**Alzheimer's Disease Edu-
cation and Referral Center**
P.O. Box 8250
Silver Spring, MD 20907
(800) 438-4380
adear@alzheimers.org

Eldercare Locator
927 15th St. NW, 6th Fl.
Washington, DC 20005
(800) 677-1116

CANCER

National Cancer Institute
(800) 4-CANCER

CHILDREN'S ISSUES

Child Molestation

Child Help USA/Child Abuse Hotline
232 East Gish Rd.
San Jose, CA 95112
(800) 422-4453

Prevent Child Abuse America
200 South Michigan Ave., Ste. 17
Chicago, IL 60604
(312) 663-3520

Crisis Intervention

Boy's Town National Hotline
(800) 448-3000

Children of the Night
P.O. Box 4343
Hollywood, CA 90078
(800) 551-1300

Covenant House Hotline
(800) 999-9999

Kid Save Line
(800) 543-7283

Youth Nineline
(referrals for parents/teens about drugs, homelessness, runaways)
(800) 999-9999

Missing Children

Missing Children...HELP Center
410 Ware Blvd., Ste. 710
Tampa, FL 33619
(800) USA-KIDS

National Center for Missing and Exploited Children
699 Prince St.
Alexandria, VA 22314
(800) 843-5678

Children with Serious Illnesses
(fulfilling wishes):

Brass Ring Society
National Headquarters
213 N. Washington St.
Snow Hill, MD 21863
(410) 632-4700
(800) 666-WISH

Make-a-Wish Foundation
(800) 332-9474

CO-DEPENDENCY

Co-Dependents
Anonymous
(602) 277-7991

DEATH/GRIEVING/
SUICIDE

Grief Recovery Institute
P.O. Box 461659
Los Angeles, CA
90046-1659
(323) 650-1234
www/grief-recovery.com

National Hospice and Palliative Care Organization
1700 Diagonal Rd., Ste. 300
Alexandria, VA 22314
(703) 243-5900
www.nhpco.org

SIDS (Sudden Infant
Death Syndrome)
Alliance
1314 Bedford Ave., Ste. 210
Baltimore, MD 21208

Parents of
Murdered Children
(recovering from violent
death of friend or family
member)
100 E 8th St., Ste. B41
Cincinnati, OH 45202
(513) 721-5683

Survivors of Suicide
Call your local Mental
Health Association for the
branch nearest you.

AARP Grief and Loss
Programs
(202) 434-2260
(800) 424-3410 ext. 2260

DEBTS

Credit Referral
(information on local credit
counseling services)
(800) 388-CCCS

Debtors Anonymous
General Service Board
P.O. Box 888

Needham, MA 02492-0009
(781) 453-2743
www.debtorsanonymous.org

DIABETES

**American Diabetes
Association**
(800) 232-3472

DOMESTIC VIOLENCE

**National Coalition
Against Domestic
Violence**
P.O. Box 34103
Washington, DC
20043-4103
(202) 745-1211

**National Domestic
Violence Hotline**
P.O. Box 161810
Austin, TX 78716
(800) 799-SAFE

DRUG ABUSE

**Cocaine Anonymous
National Referral Line**
(800) 347-8998

**National Helpline of
Phoenix House**
(cocaine abuse hotline)
(800) 262-2463
(800) COCAINE
www.drughelp.org

**National Institute of
Drug Abuse (NIDA)**
6001 Executive Blvd.,
Rm. 5213
Bethesda, MD 20892-9561
Parklawn Building
(301) 443-6245 (for information)
(800) 662-4357 (for help)

**World Service
Office, Inc. (CA)**
3740 Overland Ave., Ste. C
Los Angeles, CA
90034-6337
(310) 559-5833
(800) 347-8998 (to leave
message)

EATING DISORDERS

Overeaters Anonymous
National Office
P.O. Box 44020
Rio Rancho, NM
87174-4020
(505) 891-2664

GAMBLING

Gamblers Anonymous
New York Intergroup
P.O. Box 7
New York, NY 10116-0007
(212) 903-4400

HEALTH ISSUES

Alzheimer's Association
919 N. Michigan Ave.,
Ste. 1100
Chicago, IL 60611-1676
(800) 621-0379

**American Chronic Pain
Association**
P.O. Box 850
Rocklin, CA 95677
(916) 632-0922
www.theacpa.org

**American Foundation
of Traditional Chinese
Medicine**
P.O. Box 330267
San Francisco, CA 94133
(415) 392-7002

**American Holistic
Health Association**
P.O. Box 17400
Anaheim, CA 92817
(714) 779-6152

www.ahha.org
e-mail: ahha@healthy.net

**Chopra Center
for Well Being**
Deepak Chopra, M.D.
7630 Fay Ave.
La Jolla, CA 92037
(858) 551-7788

The Fetzer Institute
9292 West KL Ave.
Kalamazoo, MI 49009
(616) 375-2000

**Hippocrates
Health Institute**
1443 Palmdale Court
West Palm Beach, FL 33411

Hospicelink
190 Westbrook Rd.
Essex, CN 06426
(800) 331-1620

**Institute for
Noetic Sciences**
P.O. Box 909
Sausalito, CA 94966
(415) 331-5650

**The Mind-Body
Medical Institute**
110 Francis St., Ste. 1A
Boston, MA 02215
(617) 632-9525

National Health
Information Center
P.O. Box 1133
Washington, DC
20013-1133
(800) 336-4797

Optimum Health
Care Institute
6970 Central Ave.
Lemon Grove, CA 91945
(619) 464-3346

Preventive Medicine
Research Institute
Dean Ornish, M.D.
900 Bridgeway, Ste. 2
Sausalito, CA 94965
(415) 332-2525

HOUSING RESOURCES

Acorn
(nonprofit network of
low- and moderate-
income housing)
739 8th St., S.E.
Washington, DC 20003
(202) 547-9292

IMPOTENCE

Impotence Institute
of America
P.O. Box 410

Bowie, MD 20718-0410
(800) 669-1603
www.impotenceworld.org

MENTAL HEALTH

American Psychiatric
Association of America
www.psych.org

Anxiety Disorders Association of America
www.adaa.org

The Help Center of the
American Psychological
Association
www.helping.apa.org

The International Society
for Mental Health Online
www.ismho.org

Knowledge Exchange
Network
www.mentalhealth.org

National Center for Post-
Traumatic Stress Disorder
(PTSD)
www.dartmouth.edu/
dms/ptsd

National Alliance for the
Mentally Ill
www.nami.org

National Depressive
and Manic-Depressive
Association
www.ndmda.org

National Institute of
Mental Health
www.nimh.nih.gov

PET BEREAVEMENT

Bide-A-Wee Foundation
410 E. 38th St.
New York, NY 10016
(212) 532-6395

Holistic Animal
Consulting Centre
29 Lyman Ave.
Staten Island, NY 10305
(718) 720-5548

RAPE/SEXUAL ISSUES

Rape, Abuse, and Incest
National Network
(800) 656-4673

Safe Place
P.O. Box 19454
Austin, TX 78760
(512) 440-7273

National Council on
Sexual Addictions and
Compulsivity
1090 S. Northchase
Parkway, Ste. 200
South Marietta, GA 30067
(770) 989-9754

Sexually Transmitted
Disease Referral
(800) 227-8922

SMOKING

Nicotine Anonymous
P.O. Box 126338
Harrisburg, PA 17112
(415) 750-0328
www.nicotine-anony-
mous.org

STRESS REDUCTION

The Biofeedback &
Psychophysiology Clinic
The Menninger Clinic
P.O. Box 829
Topeka, KS 66601-0829
(913) 350-5000

New York Open Center
(In-depth workshops to
invigorate the spirit)
83 Spring St.
New York, NY 10012
(212) 219-2527

Omega Institute
(a healing, spiritual retreat
community)
150 Lake Dr.
Rhinebeck, NY 12572-3212
(845) 266-4444 (info)
(800) 944-1001 (to enroll)

**The Stress
Reduction Clinic**
Center for Mindfulness
University of Massachusetts
Medical Center
55 Lake Ave. North
Worcester, MA 01655
(508) 856-1616
(508) 856-2656

TEEN HELP

**ADOL: Adolescent
Directory Online**
Includes information on
eating disorders, depres-
sion, and teen pregnancy.
www.education.indiana.ed
u/cas/adol/adol.html

Al-Anon/Alateen
1600 Corporate
Landing Parkway
Virginia Beach, VA
23454-5617
(888) 425-2666
(888) 4AL-ANON
www.al-anon.org

**Focus Adolescent Services:
Eating Disorders**
www.focusas.com/
EatingDisorders.html

Future Point
A nonprofit organization
that offers message boards
and chat rooms to em-
power teens in the aca-
demic world and beyond.
www.futurepoint.org

Kids in Trouble Help Page
Child abuse, depression,
suicide, and runaway
resources, with links and
hotline numbers.
www.geocities.com/
EnchantedForest/2910

Planned Parenthood
810 Seventh Ave.
New York, NY 10019
(212) 541-7800
www.plannedparenthood.org

SafeTeens.com
Provides lessons on online safety and privacy; also has resources for homework and fun on the web.
www.safeteens.com

TeenCentral.net
This site is written by and about teens. Includes celebrity stories, real-teen tales, an anonymous help-line, and crisis counseling.
www.teencentral.net

TeenOutReach.com
Includes all kinds of infor-mation geared at teens, from sports to entertain-ment to help with drugs and eating disorders.
www.teenoutreach.com

Just for Kids Hotline
(888) 594-5437
(888) 594-KIDS

National Child Abuse Hotline
(800) 792-5200

National Runaway Hotline
(800) 621-4000

National Youth Crisis Hotline
(800) 442-4673
(800) 442-HOPE

Suicide Prevention Hotline
(800) 827-7571

Hotlines for Teenagers

**Boys Town
National Hotline**
(800) 448-3000

**Childhelp National
Child Abuse Hotline/
Voices for Children**
(800) 422-4453
(800) 4ACHILD

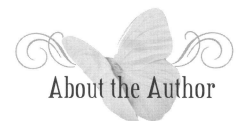

About the Author

Caroline Sutherland is an internationally recognized medical intuitive, lecturer, and workshop leader; and the author of numerous books and audiotapes on health, personal development, and self-esteem. She is the founder of Sutherland Communications, Inc., which offers medical intuitive training programs, programs for menopausal women, effective weight-loss programs, intuitive assessments, consultation services, and related products for adults and children. She is a popular guest on radio and television.

Notes

Notes

Notes

Notes

Notes

Notes

Notes

Notes

Notes